WARD LO

FAMILY HEALTH G

SPORTS
INJURIES

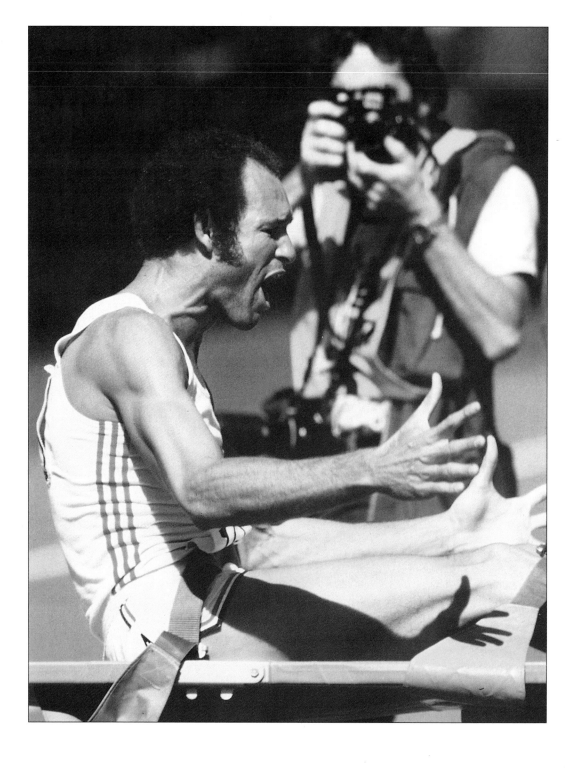

WARD LOCK

FAMILY HEALTH GUIDE

SPORTS INJURIES

DR PATRICK MILROY

IN ASSOCIATION WITH THE
NATIONAL SPORTS MEDICINE INSTITUTE

WARD LOCK

Dr Patrick Milroy
Dr Patrick Milroy is a general practitioner and Medical Advisor to the British
Athletics Federation. He has been appointed doctor to the England Athletics Team
for the 1994 Commonwealth Games and is also Medical Advisor to the UK
magazine *Runner's World*.

A WARD LOCK BOOK

First published in the UK 1994
by Ward Lock
Wellington House
125 Strand
London WC2R 0BB
A Cassell Imprint

Reprinted 1995, 1996

Designed and produced
by SP Creative Design
147 Kings Road, Bury St Edmunds, Suffolk, England
Editor: Heather Thomas
Art Director: Al Rockall
Designer: Rolando Ugolini
Illustrations: Al Rockall and Rolando Ugolini

6 17. 1027 /

Distributed in the United States
by Sterling Publishing Co., Inc.
387 Park Avenue South, New York, NY 10016-8810

A British Library Cataloguing in Publication Data
block for this book may be obtained from the British Library.

ISBN 0-7063-7253-0

Printed and bound in Spain

Acknowledgements
Cover photograph: Sporting Pictures(UK)Ltd
Mark Shearman: photos on pages, 8,9,10,11,14,15,44,52
Patrick Milroy: photos on pages, 24, 27, 29, 30, 32
The illustration on page 41 has been modified from; Lamb, D.R., 'Physiology of
Exercise, Responses and Adaptions'(Macmillan 1984)

Contents

Introduction

For whatever reason, some good some bad, the majority of the population now has more leisure time. Despite political pressures it would appear that the average life style is less and less healthy, recent statistics showing an increase for instance in both obesity and underage smoking. However, a significant proportion of the population now have both the will and the opportunity to take sporting exercise, though many would complain that campaigns labelled "Sport For All" are accompanied by injuries for all.

In no way is this intended to be a medical textbook. As such, it would be valueless to the majority of readers and could cause more harm than good. However, whilst the amount of help for the injured sportsman would by general consensus appear to be meagre, a reference book giving the basics of possible diagnosis and helpful treatments may help to restore fitness to some who would otherwise remain injured.

So it must be emphasised that this is only a guide book and any persistent or serious symptoms should always be referred for a medical opinion, preferably without any more than simple first aid initially, for a comprehensive recovery is unlikely unless a competent diagnosis has been made.

Chapter one

Injury prevention

"A stitch in time ....." runs the proverb, but the statement has similar relevance to sport and injury. There is all manner of injury which can be simply prevented by adhering to sensible practices in the areas of clothing, equipment, footwear and plain common sense. All too often this does not occur and injury results. Possibly the most important axiom to follow is that you need to be fit to play sport rather than using sport as a means of getting fit.

Training

Everybody has a baseline fitness, from those who can only walk one hundred metres without becoming short of breath, to the weekend hiker who thinks nothing of thirty miles in a day. An improvement in performance and fitness is only going to occur if the training load is modified, either by training harder or longer or more often. Whatever route is chosen any increase of more than ten per cent per week is inviting over-use injury.

Technique

This is not a coaching manual but we have all seen the naturally gifted sportsman who always appears to be graceful and co-ordinated. A player who learns proper techniques early on in his career is less likely to become injured, whilst the experienced player who knows many of the arts of the game can use these techniques to avoid injury. There is no substitute for experience, but this can only be learned slowly.

Clothing

Although many fashions appear to follow particular sports, there is often a good reason for the wearing of a special type of clothing. Sport played in summer usually requires any rise of the core body temperature to be minimized. This can be achieved with light loose fitting clothing which also allows circulation of air, reflection of the sun's rays, and absorption of sweat. However specific areas of the body may need warmth maintenance, such as the hamstrings in sprinters who often wear long cycling shorts. Dark colours retain heat and are more suitable for winter wear, though participants in long-distance stamina events need to anticipate extremes of temperature and be prepared. If in doubt it is easier to shed clothing during competition than to put it on.

Protective clothing

Out of necessity many contact sports require the participants to protect themselves against

Injury prevention

Protective clothing against heat and cold

On cold winter days it is important to keep warm. This does not mean wearing several layers of heavy clothing. Nowadays you can buy very lightweight thermal tops and jackets that allow perspiration to escape. These are ideal for runners who train in all weather conditions. They keep them warm and allow their bodies to 'breathe'. On cold days, sweat cools quickly and you may soon get cold when you drop off the pace in running or slow down in a game of soccer, and cold muscles are more susceptible to injury and stiffness.

In summer, you should opt for comfortable and practical clothing that will help take away sweat from your skin. The new Coolmax material is particularly good at this and is preferable to nylon or cotton. As a general rule, make sure that no articles of clothing are too tight, that seams are not too prominent and thereby avoid chaffing of the skin.

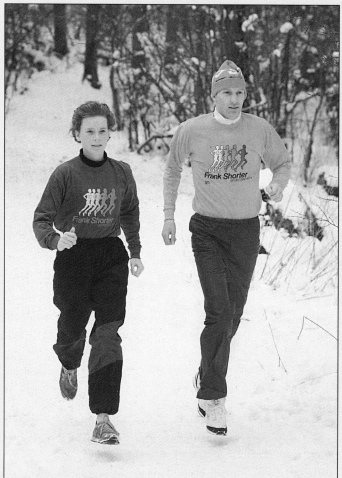

injury. Some of these items appear to be little more than fashion accessories and any protective clothing must be strong enough to prevent the player from being lulled into a false sense of security by ignoring dangerous situations, which become worse if the clothing fails in its primary task. It is equally important that protective clothing should not injure other players.

Helmets

These should be strong enough not to shatter on impact, to have a padded interior conforming to current safety standards, should not restrict neck movement, and should be held in place with soft padded straps, which can if necessary be easily removed. No player wearing a helmet should chew gum in view of the risk of inhalation and asphyxia. Any damaged helmet should be replaced immediately.

Visibility

Throughout the running boom participants have been at risk from motor vehicles. This increases ten fold at night and if wearing darkened clothing. Many shoes now have reflective tabs, but bibs and armbands of luminous material should also be *de rigeur* for the nocturnal participant.

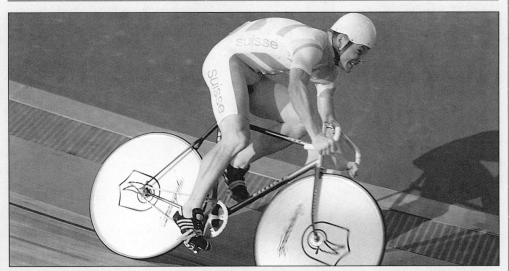

Head protection

Helmets are now worn for protection in many sports, especially American football, cricket, cycling and riding. Although they are strong enough to withstand falls and knocks, they are usually made of lightweight materials and are comfortable to wear.

Injury prevention

Eye protection

Many sports involve small flying objects and it is a paradox to imagine that it is only the hard-playing experienced exponent who becomes injured. A squash ball is theoretically interchangeable with an eyeball, so beginners especially should wear goggles, spectacles or a suitable visor when playing this form of sport. Naturally the transparent material should be unbreakable to prevent small splinters entering the eyes.

Padding

The risk with padding is that it may make the wearer feel that he is invulnerable to injury. Shoulder, shin and thigh pads will all diminish the effect of trauma to a certain extent, but they cannot prevent it completely.

Genital protector

These should not be a sporting joke. Males have been rendered infertile by trauma to the testicles and a suitably sized protector is vital.

Socks

Clean socks will not only prevent rubbing between skin and shoe, but should also be absorbent to soak up sweat and reduce the incidence of fungal infection within the feet. They should be washed regularly, as should all clothing.

The goalkeeper in hockey requires not only padded clothing but also head and face protection from the hard fast-moving ball.

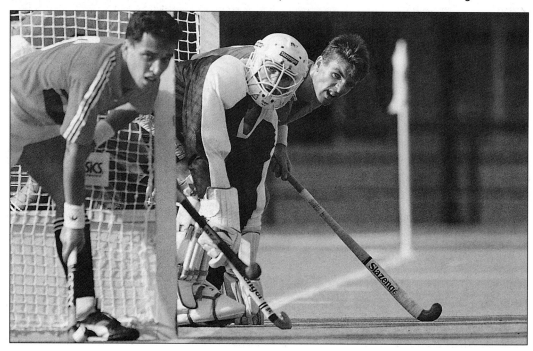

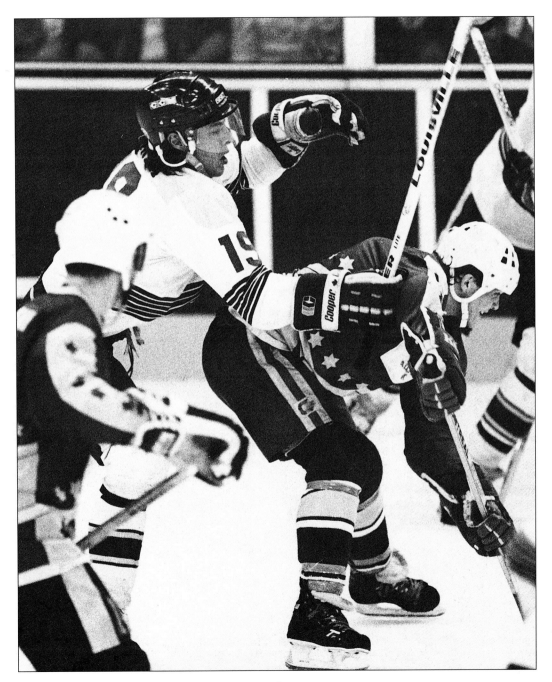

Injury prevention

Sports shoes

Any player seeking new shoes will be faced by a bewildering array of glossy and expensive footwear. The ideal shoe is one that is comfortable, flexible, hard-wearing, suitable for the sort of surface to be played on and not so expensive as to break the bank! There are, however, a few rules which should be followed in looking for shoes.

The outer sole

Whilst the runner on muddy terrain requires a good grip, which probably will employ some form of stud or waffle pattern, the road runner will prefer a softer more yielding sole where grip is less important. The player of a racket sport, where turning and changing of direction is the keynote to success, needs a sole surface which can progressively slow the player to a halt, which can prevent damage to the tendons at the front of the ankle. In some sports a sliding stop is required.

The mid sole

If the sport involves a heavy landing then plenty of padding is required. Most shoes now use artificial materials which regain their shape after compression. A football player landing on soft turf requires less mid sole padding as opposed to the road runner or hard court tennis player.

Heel counter

This is the curved heel of the shoe which supports the human anatomy. It should grip firmly, but not tightly, to prevent calcaneal bursae and bruised heel fat pads.

The uppers

These should be made of a material which allows fluid to leak in and out, to be washable, to have the minimum number of stitches and uneven areas which could cause chafing inside the shoe and to have the minimum lacing necessary to hold the shoe comfortably in place, preferably with a padded tongue. The toe box should be wide enough to permit movement and prevent toe injury. There must be enough room within the shoe for socks and an orthotic device if required, whereas there should be no heel tab if Achilles tendon problems have occurred.

Finally, feet swell during the day, so however inconvenient it may be for the shop assistant, buy your shoes half an hour before closing rather than half an hour after opening!

The illustration opposite shows the construction of a lightweight running shoe, which features heel and forefoot pads to disperse and absorb shock, a dual-density lightweight mid-sole for cushioning and lugs and a blown-rubber forefoot outsole for further cushioning and stability.

Anatomy of a sports shoe

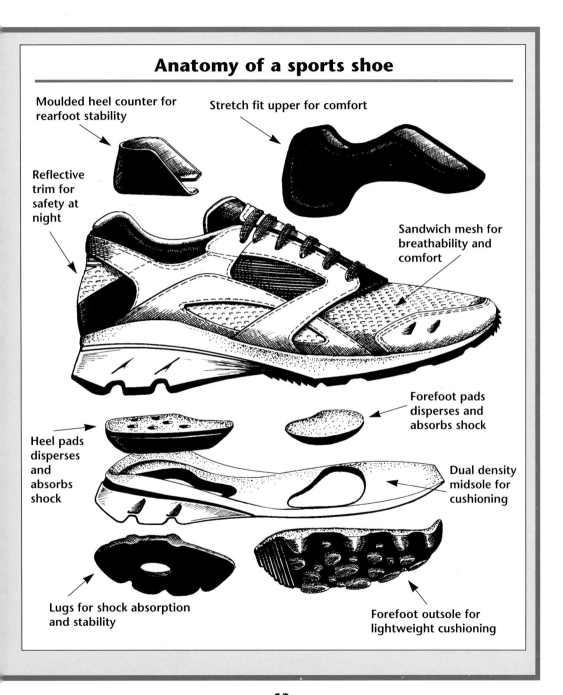

Moulded heel counter for rearfoot stability

Stretch fit upper for comfort

Reflective trim for safety at night

Sandwich mesh for breathability and comfort

Forefoot pads disperses and absorbs shock

Heel pads disperses and absorbs shock

Dual density midsole for cushioning

Lugs for shock absorption and stability

Forefoot outsole for lightweight cushioning

Injury prevention

Other forms of injury prevention

Blisters and chafing

These both occur if continued rubbing of the skin occurs. If one site is repetitively rubbed, irritation can be prevented by covering it with a plaster tape or petroleum jelly prior to the exercise.

Laws of the sport

One of the less publicized sequelae of cheating is that it may lead to injury. Although this might be thought of only as happening in combat sports, the lure of financial gain or personal advancement have led to many well publicized examples of cheating and injuries sustained therefrom. Even the runner cutting a corner may be mown down by a car that

has not been seen, a self-induced injury if ever there was one!

Other illness

It is generally unwise for a player to exercise if ill. It will certainly hinder performance and may even have fatal secondary consequences. As an example, anyone competing with a minor viral infection could develop myocarditis, which might prevent them from ever enjoying exercise again. A few days lost in recuperation is nothing in comparison to future years of enforced inactivity. Any player with a doubt as to his fitness to compete should not do so until given the go-ahead by a qualified medical practitioner.

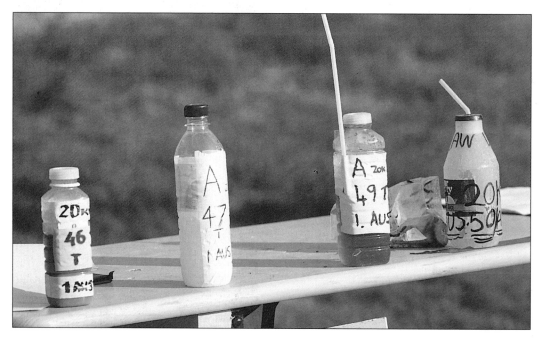

Fluids

It is a proven fact that injury is more likely when the player is dehydrated. At the other extreme, over-hydration prior to an event may lead to discomfort and stitch. Training should be used to prepare for competition, and the well trained sportsperson will have discovered long before the day of competition how much fluid he finds comfortable to drink. As relative dehydration begins immediately, it is also sensible to be prepared to drink from an early stage in any drawn-out competition requiring stamina. By the time thirst is felt, it is almost certainly too late to replace the lost fluid.

Psychology

It is natural to become nervous before competition, but an excess of adrenalin may

Fatigue

Fatigue for any reason is associated with a risk of injury. This may be due to lack of sleep or over-training, so both should be avoided.

cause an unequal distribution of effort throughout the event. Every successful sportsman has his own method of preparation, but most involve solitary concentration or meditation, warm-up, average self-confidence and a good understanding of the sport, its rules and those with whom the sportsman has contact (coaches, other team members etc.).

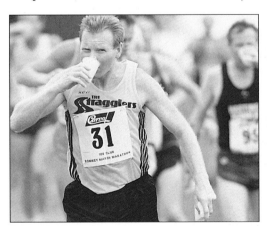

It is very important to drink when exercising in hot weather to avoid dehydration. For example, on a long-distance run, you can lose up to two litres of water in an hour just from sweating. A wet sponge will also cool the skin, and sponging stations are usually situated at three-mile intervals in many marathon races.

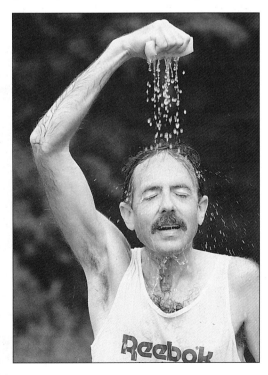

Injury prevention

Warming up

Although many sportsmen warm-up, it is often in a somewhat haphazard fashion. The first part of any warm-up should be stretching of all the relevant muscle groups. A stretch should consist of a player slowly moving a limb into a position which is just uncomfortable but never painful. It should be held for approximately thirty seconds before slowly returning to the original unstretched stance. There should never be any "rocking", which will trigger stretch reflexes within the muscle and could lead to a tear. Having stretched all the relevant muscle groups the player should then commence gentle jogging and exercising to increase metabolism and raise the heart rate. Finally a few strides at sub-maximal speed should leave the sportsman some five or ten minutes to adjust clothing and kit, visit the lavatory, and mentally prepare himself.

Neck stretches

1 Stand up straight and lift your head to look upwards.
2 Bring your head slowly forwards until your chin is resting lightly on your chest.
3 Raise your head and turn it slowly to one side. Hold the position for a few seconds.
4 Roll your head round to the other side, keeping your chin down. Hold for a few seconds. Repeat the exercise 5 times to stretch and loosen your neck.

Shoulders and arms

Above-the-head shoulder stretch

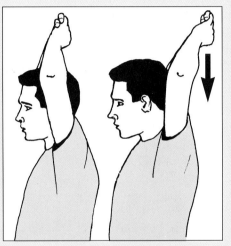

Stand up straight and raise your arms above your head, clasping your hands together. Pull them down behind you and hold for a few seconds. Repeat 5 times.

Shoulder stretch

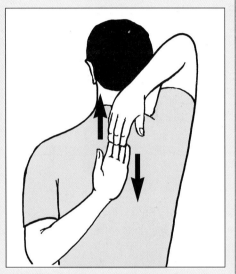

Reach down your back behind you with one hand and up with the other. Try to bring the two hands together and then pull hard in the opposite direction.

Bent arm shoulder stretch

Bend your right arm back over your head and right shoulder. Hold the elbow with your left hand and then gently pull it towards your left shoulder. Repeat the exercise on the other side.

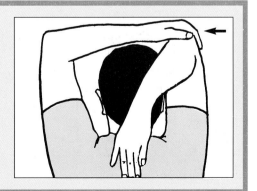

Injury prevention

The windmill

1 Stand up straight with arms hanging by your sides. Swing your right arm forwards and up and round behind you in a circle. Repeat 5 times.
2 Repeat the exercise with the left arm 5 times. If wished, you can then do the exercise again with both arms.

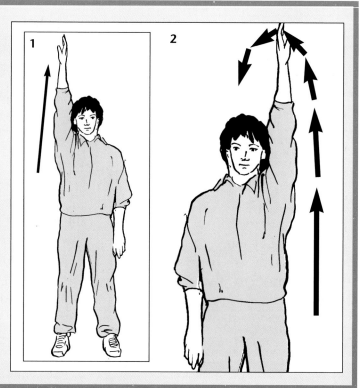

Shoulder shrugs

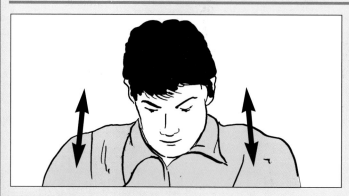

Stand up straight with your hands resting on your hips. Shrug your shoulders, rotating them slowly backwards 10 times. Then reverse and shrug them in a forwards rotation 10 times.

Triceps stretch

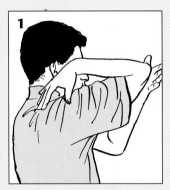 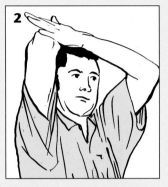 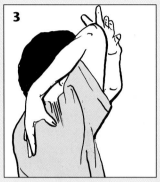

1 Stand up straight and raise your right arm with the fingertips resting on the right shoulder.

2 With your left hand, push against the right elbow.

3 Try to lower your fingers down your back as you do so. Hold for a count of 8 and then repeat on the other side.

Arm circling

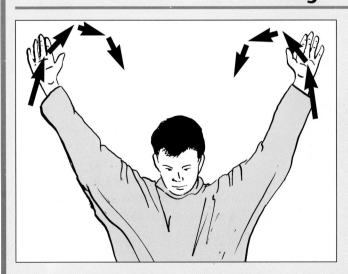

Stand up straight with your feet shoulder-width apart. Stretch your arms out to the sides at shoulder level and then circle them forwards 10 times. Repeat 10 times in a backwards motion. Make the circles as large as possible.

Injury prevention

Trunk and chest

Torso stretch

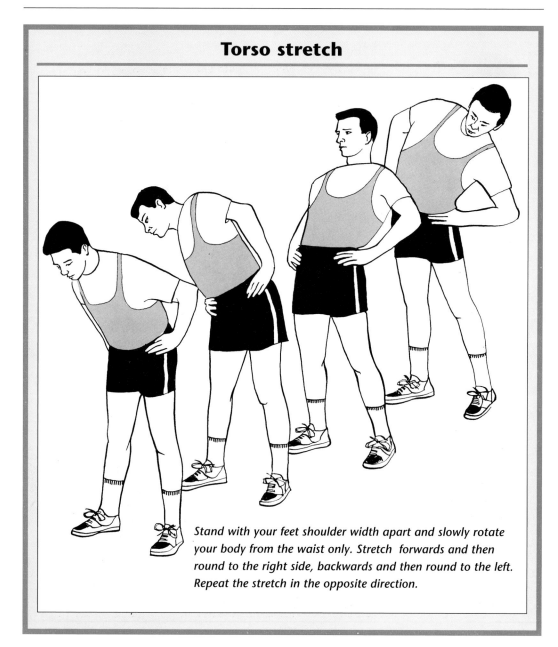

Stand with your feet shoulder width apart and slowly rotate
your body from the waist only. Stretch forwards and then
round to the right side, backwards and then round to the left.
Repeat the stretch in the opposite direction.

Trunk rotations

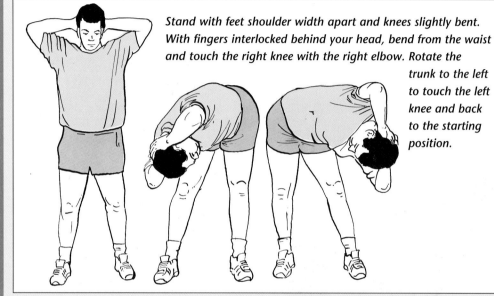

Stand with feet shoulder width apart and knees slightly bent. With fingers interlocked behind your head, bend from the waist and touch the right knee with the right elbow. Rotate the trunk to the left to touch the left knee and back to the starting position.

Trunk turns

Stand with feet apart and knees slightly bent. Raise your arms to shoulder height and clasp your hands. Turn from the waist to one side as far as you can go. Hold for a count of 5 and then turn to the other side. Keep your legs and hips still and turn only the upper body.

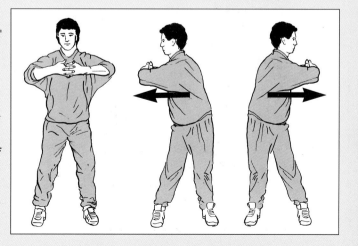

Injury prevention

Side bends

Stand up straight with hands by your sides and knees slightly bent. Slowly raise one arm high above your head, easing the other arm down your leg. Pull your arm over your head as far as it will go while pushing down on your thigh. Return to the starting position and repeat on the other side. Do 3 repetitions on each side.

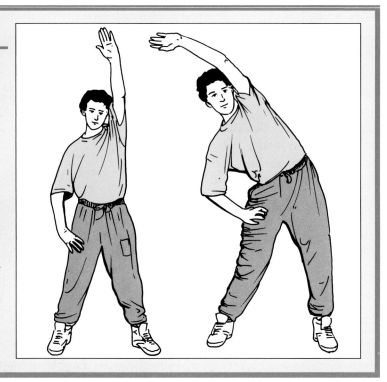

Chest flings

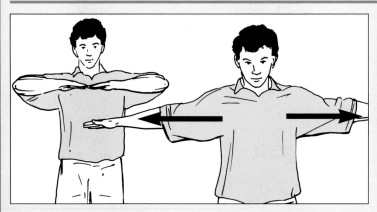

Stand up straight with feet shoulder width apart, elbows bent at shoulder height and fingertips touching. Fling your arms out gently backwards at shoulder height and then return to the original position. Repeat 10 times.

Back

Upper back stretch

Stand up straight with your hands clasped together behind your back. Lift them upwards and outwards as high as possible. Hold for a count of 5 and then lower them to the starting position. Repeat 5 times.

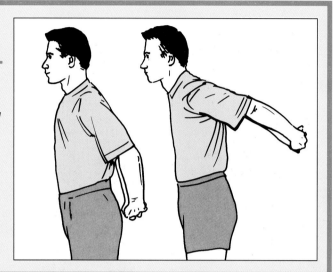

Alternative upper back stretch

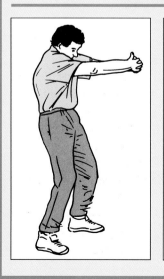

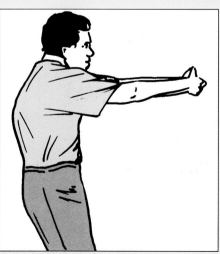

Stand with feet shoulder width apart and knees slightly bent. Interlock your fingers and raise your arms to shoulder height. Push your arms forwards without leaning forwards. Hold the stretch for a count of 10. Repeat 5 times.

Injury prevention

Lower back stretch

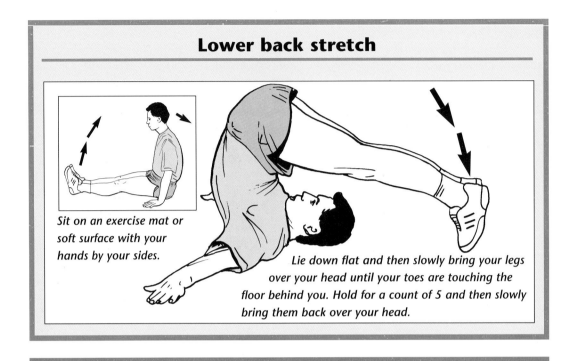

Sit on an exercise mat or soft surface with your hands by your sides.

Lie down flat and then slowly bring your legs over your head until your toes are touching the floor behind you. Hold for a count of 5 and then slowly bring them back over your head.

Lumbar stretch

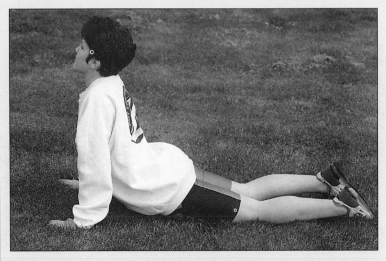

Lie on the ground and raise your upper body supporting your weight with your hands, palms flat on the ground as shown. Keeping your arms straight, stretch gently upwards, raising your head and chin. Repeat 3 times.

Hips and groin

Side stretch

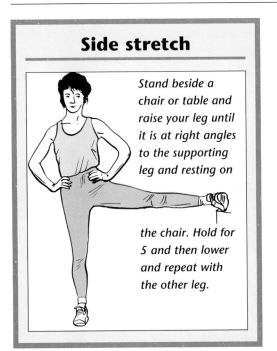

Stand beside a chair or table and raise your leg until it is at right angles to the supporting leg and resting on

the chair. Hold for 5 and then lower and repeat with the other leg.

Knee flex

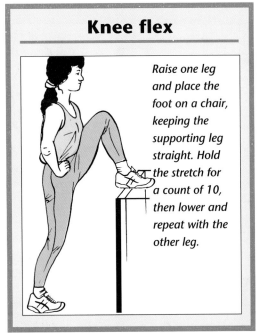

Raise one leg and place the foot on a chair, keeping the supporting leg straight. Hold the stretch for a count of 10, then lower and repeat with the other leg.

Ski stretch

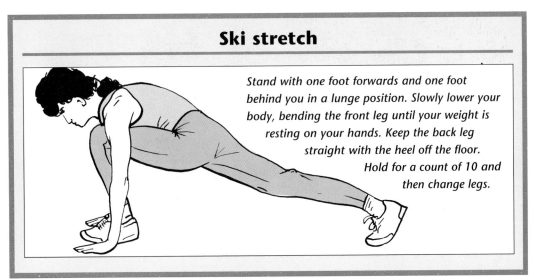

Stand with one foot forwards and one foot behind you in a lunge position. Slowly lower your body, bending the front leg until your weight is resting on your hands. Keep the back leg straight with the heel off the floor. Hold for a count of 10 and then change legs.

Injury prevention

Hip rotations

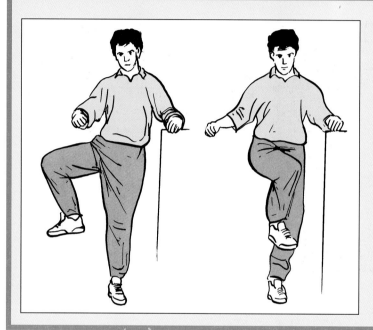

Stand holding on to a rail or the back of a chair and lift and bend one knee. Push the bent knee across your body to touch the opposite hip. Repeat 10 times and then repeat with the other leg.

Groin stretch

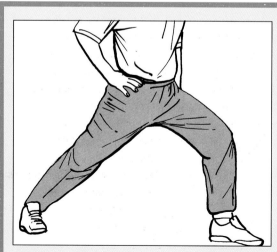

Stand up straight and place one leg about one stride in front of the other. With your hands resting lightly on your hips, bend the front leg, transferring your weight on to it. Keep your back leg straight and hold for a count of 5. Repeat 5 times with each leg.

Adductors

Adductors stretch

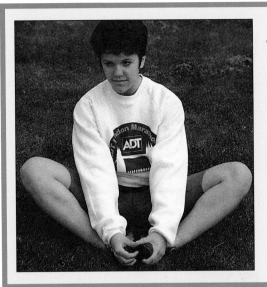

Sit on the ground with the soles of your feet pressed together and clasp your feet in your hands. Gently try to lower your knees towards the floor, leaning forwards from the hips. You will feel the stretch in your adductors.

Adductor stretch

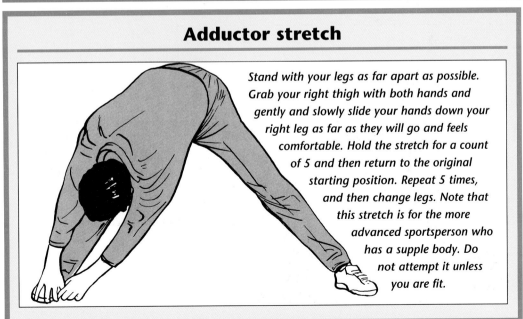

Stand with your legs as far apart as possible. Grab your right thigh with both hands and gently and slowly slide your hands down your right leg as far as they will go and feels comfortable. Hold the stretch for a count of 5 and then return to the original starting position. Repeat 5 times, and then change legs. Note that this stretch is for the more advanced sportsperson who has a supple body. Do not attempt it unless you are fit.

Injury prevention

Gluteal stretch

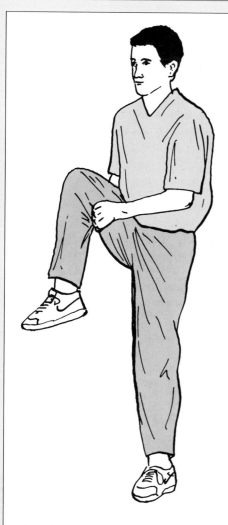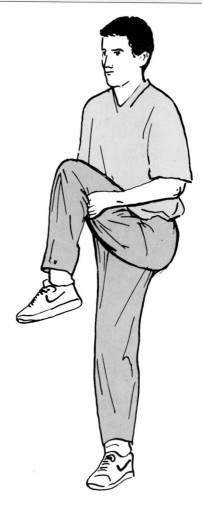

Standing up straight, raise your right leg and interlock your hands under your raised knee. Hold for a count of 10.

Lower your leg and then repeat on the other side. Do 3 repetitions each side.

Hamstrings

Hamstring stretch

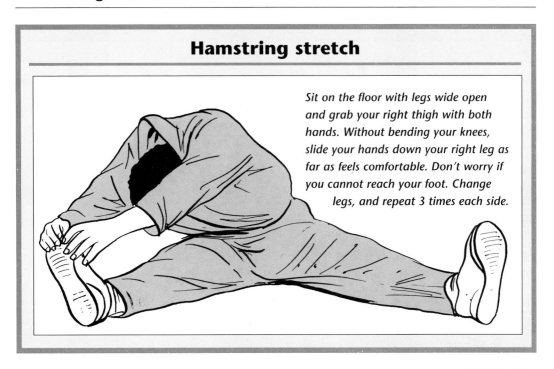

Sit on the floor with legs wide open and grab your right thigh with both hands. Without bending your knees, slide your hands down your right leg as far as feels comfortable. Don't worry if you cannot reach your foot. Change legs, and repeat 3 times each side.

Alternative hamstring stretch

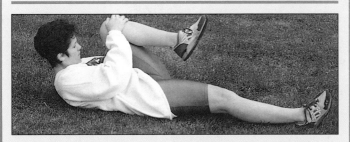

Lie on your back and raise one leg off the ground with the knee bent. Raise your head and shoulders off the ground and clasp your knee in both hands, gently pulling it in towards your chest. Repeat on the other side.

Important

You should stretch your hamstrings only as far as feels comfortable. Do not touch your toes unless you are really fit and supple.

Injury prevention

Raised hamstring stretch

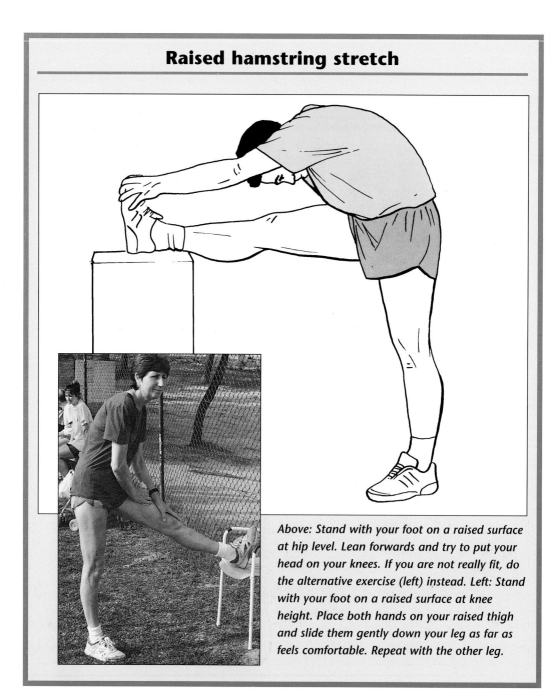

Above: Stand with your foot on a raised surface at hip level. Lean forwards and try to put your head on your knees. If you are not really fit, do the alternative exercise (left) instead. Left: Stand with your foot on a raised surface at knee height. Place both hands on your raised thigh and slide them gently down your leg as far as feels comfortable. Repeat with the other leg.

Hamstring stretch

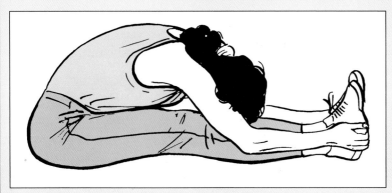

Again, you should only do this if you are very fit. Sit down with legs outstretched and close together. Slowly bend forwards from the hips and clasp your feet in your hands.

Hurdler's hamstring stretch

Sit down with one leg stretched out in front and the other leg bent at the knee at 90 degrees to the body. Lean slowly forwards from the hips, sliding your hands down your outstretched leg as far as feels comfortable. Repeat on the other side.

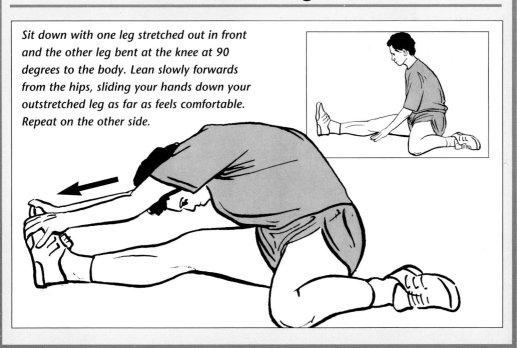

Injury prevention

Quadriceps

Quadriceps stretch

Kneel with one knee on the ground and the other bent in front of you with your foot flat on the ground. Raise the foot behind you as far as it will go and clasp it in both hands as shown. Hold the stretch for a few seconds, then lower your foot, and repeat to the other side.

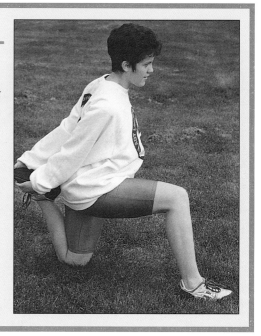

Sitting quadriceps stretch

Kneel with your toes pointing backwards away from the body behind you. Slowly lean back with your hands placed on your feet and lifting the pelvis up and out. repeat 5 times.

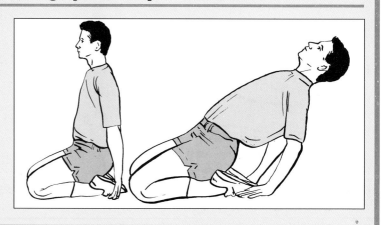

Quadriceps stretch

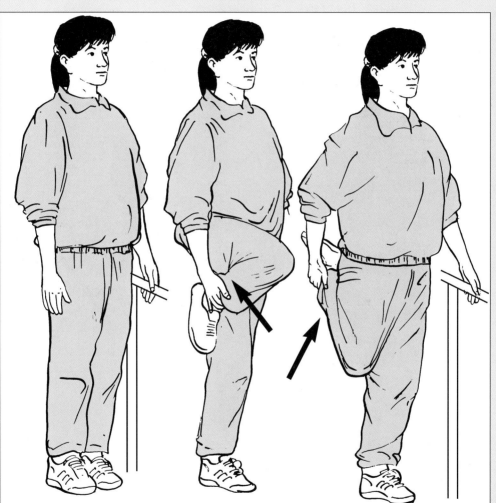

Stand up holding on to a bar or chair back, feet shoulder width apart. Raise your right knee and grasp your right ankle in your right hand. Take your leg back until the heel is close to your bottom. Hold for a count of 10 and repeat with the other leg. Be sure to keep the knees together when you take your leg back.

Injury prevention

Calf muscles

Calf stretch

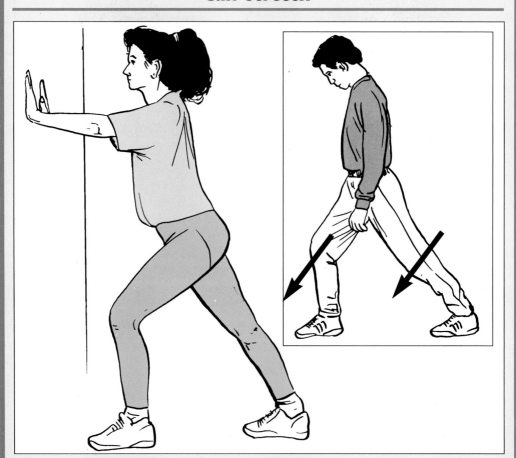

Stand up straight facing a wall with the knee nearest the wall bent and the other leg straight behind you. Place your hands on the wall and lean slowly forwards, keeping your feet flat on the ground. Hold for a few seconds and then repeat on the other side. Do 3 repetitions. Alternatively you can do the stretch in a standing position with slightly bent knees (above right). Bend forwards at the knees, keeping the heels flat on the ground.

Calf stretch

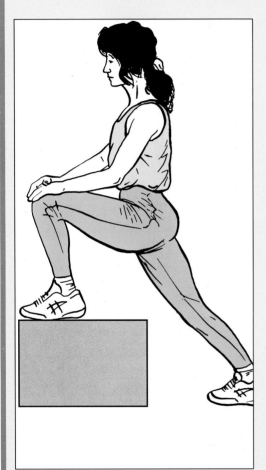

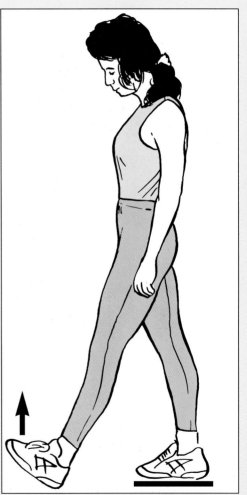

Above: Stand with one leg raised, knee bent and foot resting on a bench or stool at knee height. Make sure that the whole foot is on the bench with the heel down. Press down on your bent knee with both hands and hold the stretch for a count of 10. Repeat with the other leg.

Above: Stand up straight with one leg about 12 inches in front of the other. Raise the toes of the forward foot as far as possible. Keep the heel on the ground and hold for a count of 10. Repeat with the other leg.

Injury prevention

Alternative stretch – bent knees

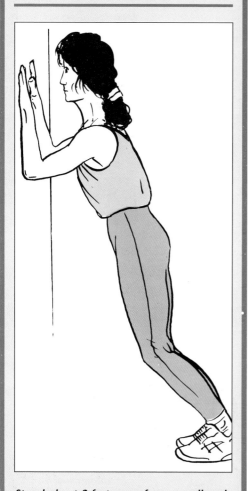

Stand about 2 feet away from a wall and lean against it with the knees slightly bent. Keep your heels flat on the floor and feel the stretch in the calf muscles. Hold for a count of 10. Do 3 repetitions.

Calf stretch

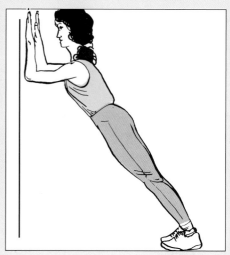

Stand about 4 feet away from a wall with your toes slightly turned in, legs together and lean against it, keeping your feet flat on the ground. Hold for a count of 10. Repeat the stretch 3 times.

Warming down

After completing his activity, the tired sportsman will frequently neglect this important part of competition. By jogging for ten minutes and slowly reducing the heart rate, less lactic acid will build up in the tissues and stiffness can be reduced. This should be done in warm clean clothes and in your training footwear. A shower and gentle stretching during the hours before bed will help you feel fresher the next day.

Chapter two

Classification of injuries

Sports injuries may be classified in a variety of different ways. Many injuries are sport dependent, but the simplest classification divides those from external forces into one group and those due to over-use or internal forces into another group of injuries. However it is necessary to understand basic anatomy of the musculo-skeletal system before describing injuries that can occur to each type of structure.

The human body

● **Bones** are the structural scaffolding of the body and are joined to other bones through synovial joints.

● **Synovial joints** are lubricated with synovial fluid contained within a capsule to allow movement. The movement may be contained by the structure of the bones or by flexible, if inelastic, connective tissue.

● **Ligaments** limit any abnormal movement. The movement between two bones is facilitated by groups of muscles which alternately contract and expand when stimulated by input from the nerves within the central nervous system.

● **Muscles** themselves are usually attached to bone through tendons which are much stronger and thinner than muscle and allow muscle pull to be concentrated through a small space such as at the wrist.

● **Bursas** are fluid sacs that prevent friction between two moving surfaces within the

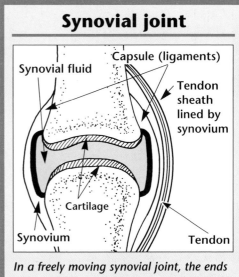

Synovial joint

In a freely moving synovial joint, the ends of the bones are encased in a capsule and ligaments. The joint is lubricated by synovial fluid secreted by the synovial membrane; this helps prevent friction.

Classification of injuries

The human skeleton

Skull

Jaw

Clavicle (collar bone

Scapula (shoulder blade)

Sternum
(Breast bone)

Ribs

Humerus

Spine

Radius

Ulna

Pelvis

Carpals
(wrist bones)

Metacarpals
(palm bones)

Phalanges
(finger bones)

Femur (thigh bone)

Patella (knee cap)

Tibia (shin bone)

Fibula

Tarsals (ankle bones)

Metatarsals
(foot bones)

Phalanges
(toe bones)

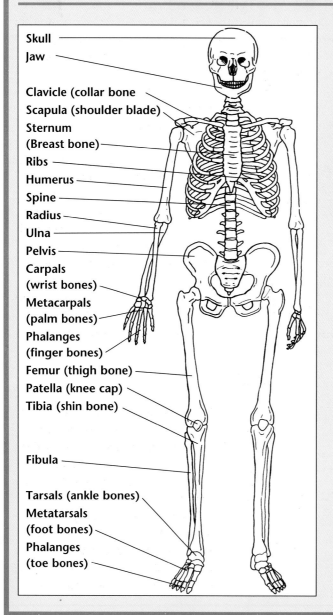

Your skeleton gives your body its shape and supports and protects it. There are 206 bones in the skeleton, which are made of living matter and are constantly being replaced with new material by their cells. The skeleton forms the structural scaffolding of the body. The bones are joined to each other through synovial joints.

body. However, if rubbed they becomes inflamed and full of fluid producing a condition known as a bursitis.

Any external and many over-use internal injuries show as either a macro or microscopic tear with disruption of the surrounding blood vessels and other soft tissues. The greater the amount of bleeding the longer the injury is likely to take to heal, so any steps to minimize this are welcome. A guide to memorize this is the following mnemonic:

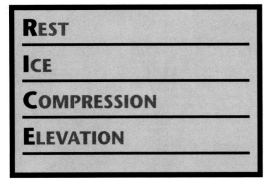

REST

ICE

COMPRESSION

ELEVATION

Ice should be wrapped in a soft, damp cloth and applied to the injury for no more than fifteen minutes at a time, though this can be repeated every hour. Compression acts as a counter pressure to blood leaking from the damaged vessels, but should not be so tight as to restrict arterial blood flow. Elevation reduces the pressure within the leaking blood vessels when the injured limb is higher than the heart.

If there is any suspicion whatsoever that a bone may be broken, especially when used for weight bearing, then the patient should be transferred to hospital for an X-ray and further treatment. If an ambulance is not available the lower limbs should be splinted together using a piece of wood with soft padding between hard surfaces, and the patient lifted carefully in and out of the vehicle. If a fracture has occurred, long bones are likely to need to be immobilized for twelve weeks or so, and a shorter bone for

Ice packs

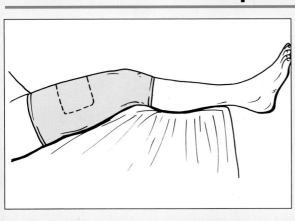

When applying an ice pack, the injured limb should be elevated to reduce the pressure within the leaking blood vessels. The ice should be wrapped in a soft, damp cloth which has been wrung out in cold water. It is important that you apply the ice for no more than 15 minutes maximum. Leaving it on for longer will be detrimental rather than helpful. If you can't get ice, use frozen peas instead.

Classification of injuries

approximately half that time. Any attempt to use the bone too soon may lead to non-union of the fracture.

Far more commonly, bones are bruised. The pain that is felt is the result of lifting of the layer of periosteum which lines the bone and bleeding between these layers. This bruise, or haematoma, often cannot escape and takes a long time to be reabsorbed. Most people have an irregular bony surface along the front of their shins, often caused by childhood trauma to the periosteum.

Stress fractures

A stress fracture is somewhat akin to a crack in a china cup as the bone is technically broken but is held together by surface tension and surrounding tissues. It is the result of repetitive movement and it is characterized by increasing or crescendo pain the more the movement is repeated. Diagnosis is not always simple and may require X-rays and bone scans, but the player who ignores these symptoms of increasing pain is liable to end up with a complete fracture. Treatment does not necessarily require the use of immobilization and plaster of Paris, but avoidance of the exercise that provokes the pain should be for three to four weeks in a short bone, six to eight in a long bone.

Muscles

Skeletal muscle consists of long bundles of fibres which contract and shorten, so bringing the attachments at each end together. Each bundle of fibres is contained within a tissue sheath, groups of these forming a named muscle. Muscles tend to have a very good

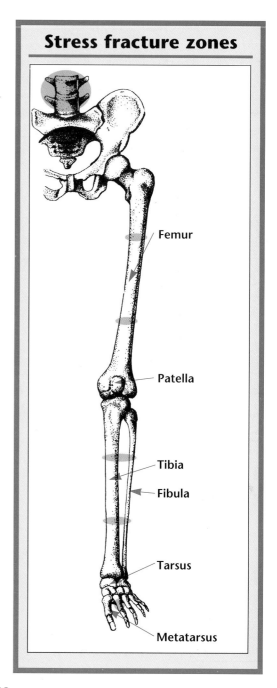

Stress fracture zones

Femur

Patella

Tibia

Fibula

Tarsus

Metatarsus

Structure of a muscle

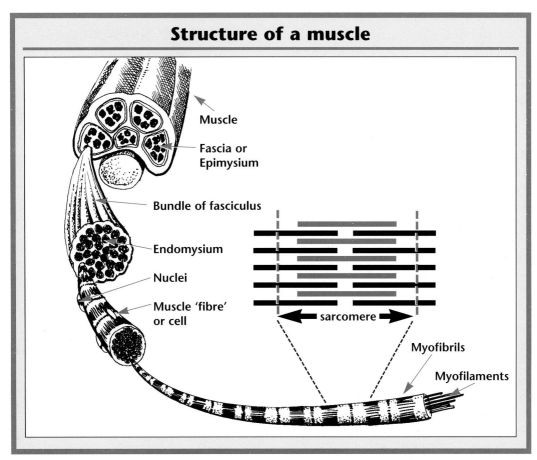

Muscle

Fascia or Epimysium

Bundle of fasciculus

Endomysium

Nuclei

Muscle 'fibre' or cell

sarcomere

Myofibrils

Myofilaments

The illustration above shows the structure of skeletal muscle.

blood supply, so bleed profusely if injured. Injuries may be classified in two ways.

1 Complete tears

Complete rupture of a muscle may cause profuse bleeding and look horrific, leaving two bumps and a gap between the torn ends. Amazingly this rarely causes much disability as other muscles take over the lost function.

Surgical repair is not required, although sensible retraining of other muscles is.

2 Partial tears

Where the rupture includes part of the muscle bundle sheath, blood is able to escape from the site of injury so although there may be much visible evidence of bruising, the effects are minimized and healing will occur within a couple of weeks if the RICE regime is followed.

With an intramuscular tear the waste blood and tissue fluid cannot escape, and an

Classification of injuries

intramuscular haematoma forms which is painful and tender, causing much limitation of movement. Treatment again requires RICE, but after forty eight hours, regulated and increasing active movement is vital to prevent stiffening and scarring within the muscle. Physiotherapy is very helpful.

If the haematoma is not mobilized scar tissue will form. This is inelastic and will lead to the muscle healing 'short'. Full stretching of the limb at warm-up thus not only helps to prevent this type of injury, but also ensures its non-recurrence.

Occasionally the blood cannot escape and calcification occurs within the muscle haematoma producing a condition called Myositis ossificans. This is worsened by over-enthusiastic mobilization, so any bruising within muscle which becomes hard and very tender must be treated gently as treatment will certainly require physiotherapy and occasionally surgery. This injury may take many months to heal.

Tendons

The tendons that join muscle to bone are composed of bundles of collagen fibres. Tendons are surrounded by a soft tissue paratenon and most of the injuries are due either to over-use or sudden stretching.

The back of leg miuscles   *(hamstring)*

1 *Gluteus medius*
2 *Gluteus maximus*
3 *Iliotibial tract*
4 *Adductor magnus*
5 *Semitendinosus*

6 *Biceps femoris*
  (hamstrings)
7 *Sartorius*
8 *Gastrocnemius*
9 *Soleus*

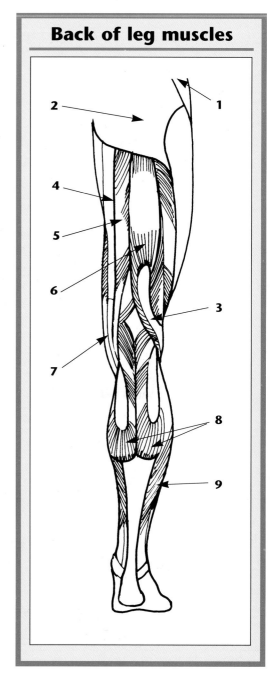

Back of leg muscles

Complete and partial rupture of achilles tendon

Complete rupture

This can happen so suddenly and noisily that the victim may imagine that he has been shot. The Achilles tendon and biceps are most commonly affected and naturally there is no function following the injury.

Bleeding occurs between the split ends, which can fill with blood, clot and in the non-sportsman be allowed to heal within a plaster of Paris casing (for the Achilles tendon). However, it is generally considered that most sportsmen regain better function if the injury is surgically repaired.

Partial rupture

These are common and although these can on occasions be returned to full activity solely through the use of physiotherapy, many sufferers require surgical excision of the scar tissue at some time in the future.

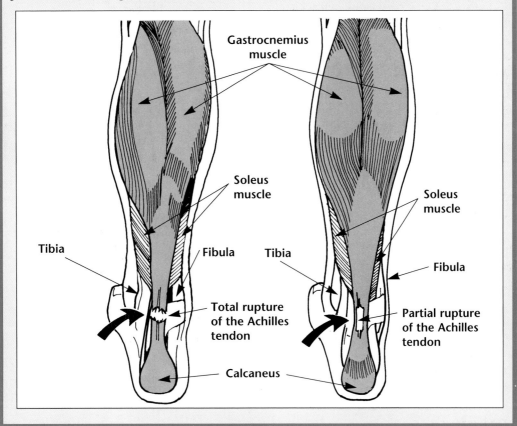

Gastrocnemius muscle

Soleus muscle

Soleus muscle

Tibia

Fibula

Tibia

Fibula

Total rupture of the Achilles tendon

Partial rupture of the Achilles tendon

Calcaneus

Classification of injuries

Simple tendinitis

This produces considerable local discomfort but with little swelling and is often the result of sudden unaccustomed exertion. The majority of players who remember RICE will recover rapidly.

Peritendinitis

Over-use of the tendon may well induce an inflammation in the surrounding paratenon, known as a peritendinitis. This will cause the area to swell, become tender and may exhibit the medical sign known as crepitus, where movement of the tendon causes a crackling sensation under any palpating fingers. Treatment may be with anti-inflammatory medication on top of RICE, but steroid injections are sometimes required provided that they are not injected into the tendon itself, a not uncommon cause of rupture!

Women in sport

There is no reason why women should not enjoy sport as much as their male counterparts. Certain problems may occur:

1 Pre-menstrual problems Weight gain and mood and concentration impairment may all affect performance. In certain women it may prove possible to delay periods using progesterone hormones or decrease the premenstrual symptoms by the use of vitamin B6 or the contraceptive pill.

2 Amenorrhoea Sportswomen undertaking heavy training may find that their periods become lighter or disappear completely. There are various mechanisms for this, though the periods usually return when the training load is lightened. This amenorrhoea does not prevent pregnancy!

3 Menstrual periods These may be irregular as a result of the stress of competition, though some women claim to compete better whilst menstruating. Internal tampons prevent personal embarrassment, but the periods may be delayed with hormones until competition is over.

4 Pregnancy There is no reason why a pregnant woman should not indulge in sport providing that she does not exhaust herself.

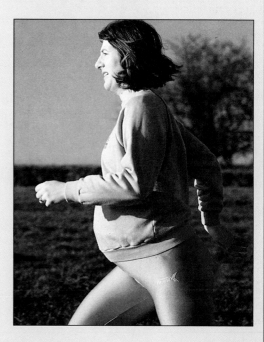

Chapter three

Upper body injuries

So far as the layman is concerned all head and neck injuries are serious until proved otherwise. While some injuries occur more or less deliberately in contact sports, others are accidental and may range from a simple bleeding laceration to death from brain damage. Intermediate states may include concussion with amnesia or coma. Apart from a surface laceration, the safe course with any head injury is immediate referral for assessment in the Accident and Emergency department of the nearest hospital. This is even more pressing if the patient appears vague or disorientated.

Here a full assessment can take place. X-rays can be ordered and if the patient is considered fit enough to return home, he should do so preferably in the company of a responsible adult with a printed head injury instruction card.

Return to sport should not be allowed until the player has been well rested and assessed to exclude post-traumatic syndrome. This may well be from three to four weeks, and in certain sports, such as rugby union, the player is banned by the laws of the sport from playing for a specified time. This is a sensible precaution although it may be resented.

Neck and spinal injuries

Falls off horses, rugby scrums and diving into shallow water can all produce spinal injury. The injured player may be conscious or unconscious. First aid in the unconscious head or neck injured player requires the following action (see page 46):

If these are satisfactory the player should not be moved until specialist help is at hand to prevent worsening the injury. Eye injuries are not uncommon. It is usually inappropriate to attempt to treat them at the site of injury and they should be viewed by a specialist in a hospital.

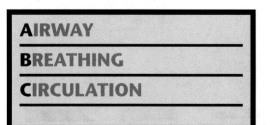

AIRWAY

BREATHING

CIRCULATION

First aid

It is always useful to have a basic knowledge of first aid. Find out about courses in your area.

Upper body injuries

ABC of resuscitation

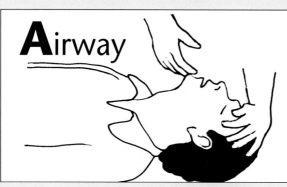

Airway

There must be a clear airway to allow oxygenated air to reach the lungs. You can gently tilt the head and lift the chin to pull the tongue clear of the airway. Take care if you suspect neck injuries.

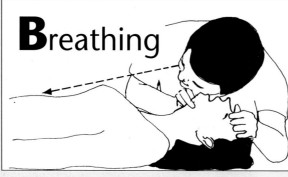

Breathing

The patient must be breathing so that the blood in the lungs can be replenished with oxygen. You should look, listen and feel for signs of breathing. If the casualty is not breathing, you should perform mouth-to-mouth ventilation after checking the carotid pulse(below).

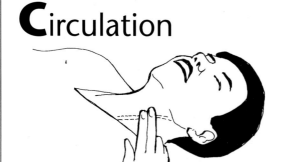

Circulation

The circulation of blood must be effective in order to distribute oxygen around the casualty's body. If you cannot detect breathing, you will need to locate the carotid pulse in the neck to check the circulation.

The upper limbs

Although muscles within the upper limbs can be injured and require treatment with RICE and rehabilitation in the usual way, it is the joints that cause problems from their variable designs.

The principal shoulder joint is inherently unstable, for although the bony components permit a wide range of movement, this mechanism also permits many injuries. The structure of the joint is maintained by four major muscles and several other minor ones producing the rotator cuff (see below).

Shoulder injuries

If the upper arm is forced out of its socket by a fall or wrenching action, it commonly dislocates in a forward direction. Pain will usually be present and the patient is unable to move his arm outwards.

Observation will show asymmetry with the other shoulder. As it is possible to sustain a fracture of the humerus at the same time, it is important not to attempt to reduce the dislocation at the time of occurrence and send the player back on the field, but to have the injury viewed where X-rays can be obtained.

The loosening effect of the dislocation means that for some people the dislocation

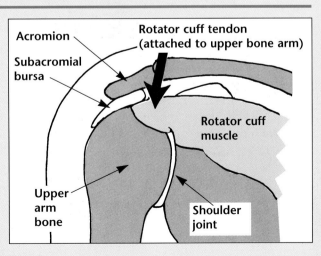

Rotator cuff

This illustration of the shoulder joint region shows the rotator cuff, a group of small muscles and tendons which are attached to the upper arm bone and hold it in the shoulder socket. The tendons may be torn or oven ruptured by sudden forceful injuries, whereas repetitive movements in throwing and racket sports, swimming and weight-lifting can all cause swelling and inflammation.

Acromion

Subacromial bursa

Rotator cuff tendon (attached to upper bone arm)

Rotator cuff muscle

Upper arm bone

Shoulder joint

may become recurrent, and may require surgery. Once a dislocation has been reduced and healing has occurred the player should gradually build up the strength of all the muscles of the rotator cuff using a series of graduated exercises. The player is reliant upon the power of these muscles to keep the shoulder in place and for future throwing or pulling strength.

Painful arc

Over-use of the shoulder muscles may result in pain as the upper arm is moved outwards in the range above and below the horizontal. Because the sufferer finds it exquisitely painful and avoids movement, there is further limit to

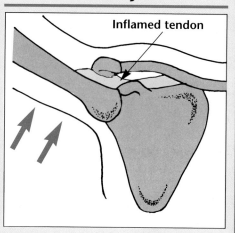

Frozen joint

Inflamed tendon

This is characterized by a painful, stiff shoulder and is another over-use injury. The lining of the shoulder joint becomes inflamed. This condition often affects middle-aged sportspeople.

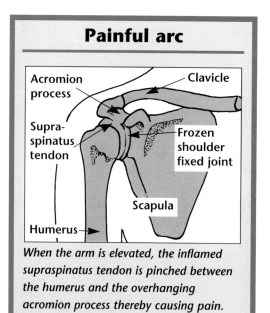

Painful arc

Acromion process

Clavicle

Supra-spinatus tendon

Frozen shoulder fixed joint

Scapula

Humerus

When the arm is elevated, the inflamed supraspinatus tendon is pinched between the humerus and the overhanging acromion process thereby causing pain. This over-use injury affects players in contact sports, throwers, racket players and weight-lifters.

the range. Early treatment with physiotherapy, massage and sometimes a steroid injection will minimize the disability and prevent chronic pain affecting the player which is known to last for many months or years.

Frozen shoulder

This describes the condition where the shoulder is 'frozen' after some form of over-use. Initially it is most comfortable to rest the shoulder, but a loading dose of anti-inflammatory drugs, ice and mobilization under the guidance of a physiotherapist should limit the time to recovery. In many cases this may take a long time in spite of all the therapies that medicine has to offer.

Subacromial bursa

Pain occurs in the shoulder when the arm is brought overhead as for throwing or swimming. The bursa under the bony acromion is trapped and will need treatment with anti-inflammatory drugs, a steroid injection and physiotherapy. Training may have to be reduced for the swimmer, and techniques changed in the throwing sports.

Acromio-clavicular joint pain

This joint between the collar bone and the top of the shoulder can be sprained by a fall which leaves an appearance as though there is a 'step' at the top of the shoulder. If it has been sprained it should be allowed to heal whilst well strapped with the elbow in a sling for an unstable A-C joint will severely limit the strength in the associated limb.

Subacromial bursitis

Acromion process

In this condition the bursa is trapped under the acromion process when the arm is lifted. It commonly affects throwers and swimmers.

The biceps muscle

Two injuries may affect this muscle at the front of the upper arm.They are:

Biceps tendinitis

Where the long head of biceps passes through a groove in the humerus (upper arm bone) inflammation can occur which is painful and can prevent throwing or which causes pain when putting the arm into the sleeve of a coat. Testing for this injury can be performed by opposing elbow bending which will cause pain. If physiotherapy and anti-inflammatories fail to settle the condition, a cortisone injection may be successful.

Rupture of long head of biceps

This can occur in vigorous sports such as weight-lifting and causes a swelling such as that associated with the cartoon character 'Popeye'. Although this looks alarming, other upper arm muscles can perform the same task, and after mobilization and rehabilitation there is usually little if any loss of strength, though the deformity is all too evident.

Upper body injuries

Rupture of biceps

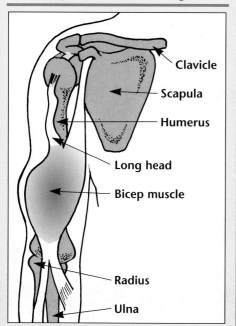

Clavicle

Scapula

Humerus

Long head

Bicep muscle

Radius

Ulna

Vigorous lifting and canoeing can cause inflammation of the biceps muscle or even rupture as shown here. This is not as alarming as it looks and can usually be treated by physiotherapy without the need for surgical repair.

Tennis elbow

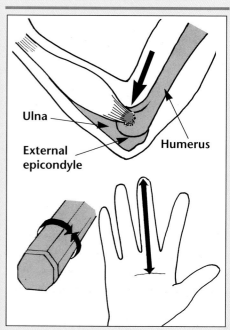

Ulna

External epicondyle

Humerus

This injury is not confined to tennis players. However, they can help relieve the pain by enlarging the circumference of the racket handle. It should be equal to the distance from the first crease in the palm to the tip of the middle finger

Elbow injuries

Tennis elbow (lateral epicondylitis)

The pain found on the outside of the elbow is commonly caused by sports in which the wrist is over-used. Despite the name this is less commonly tennis as this sport involves the whole arm with relatively little wrist movement. The over-use produces pain at the origin of the muscles that extend the wrist at the lower outer end of the humerus. The over-stretching causes pain, inflammation and

Diagnosing tennis elbow

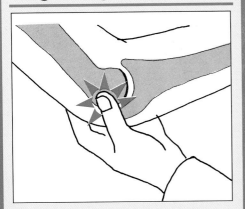

Tenderness in the bony area of the elbow is a sign of tennis elbow. Symptoms range from mild discomfort when the arm is used to severe pain, which increases when making gripping or twisting movements.

classic discomfort when opening doors or pouring from a teapot. Many "do-it-yourself" jobs induce the pain. Because it is an inflammation, RICE is the first line of treatment, but may not prevent recurrence.

The sufferer will find that the tighter he grips the handle of his racket, the worse the pain, so help may be obtained by enlarging the circumference of the racket handle. Ideally this circumference should be the same as from the first crease in the palm to the tip of the middle finger. Poor technique or a heavy racket, which the player is unable to control may also be implicated. If rest fails to resolve the pain, a steroid injection is often given, but movement of the injured muscle can also be limited by a strapping one inch wide round the upper forearm, which may still allow play.

At home it may help to stretch the arm in a fixed position, elbow straight, forearm turned in, wrist bent forward and held by the other hand. This gentle discomfort should be maintained for thirty seconds or so and repeated as often as is practical.

Golfer's elbow

This is the equivalent condition which can affect the muscles originating from the inner side of the elbow. It is less common than tennis elbow and is frequently associated with a poor technique and hitting divots! The same practical treatments apply except that to stretch the damaged muscles, the wrist should be pulled backwards, though the best advice may well be a lesson from the professional!

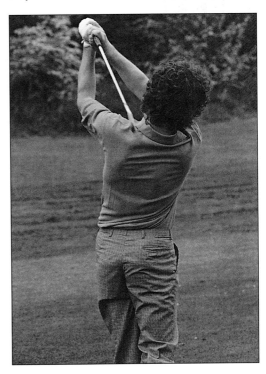

Upper body injuries

Thrower's elbow

This condition particularly affects athletes such as javelin throwers and cricketers who have to extend the elbow to its fullest extent. This imposes stress on the inner side of the elbow where a ligament can be partially torn away and if allowed to continue unchecked may well finish the thrower's career through an inability to fully extend the elbow. A combination of good coaching, reduced training, physiotherapy and a steroid injection can alleviate the condition, though in many cases treatment is unavailing.

Tenosynovitis of the forearm

Although presenting in various ways, this painful condition of the muscles of the forearm usually causes swelling and discomfort on movement of the wrist or fingers. It is the result of over-use of these muscles, especially where there are rapid repeated wrist movements such as in gymnastics or rowing. Examination produces pain if contraction of the muscles is resisted, and there is often a crackling sensation felt as these muscles are moved. Treatment by anti-inflammatories, RICE, and cessation of the provoking action may relieve the condition, but once again steroid injections can produce a rapid reduction of symptoms. As poor technique may have caused the original injury, good coaching can prevent recurrence.

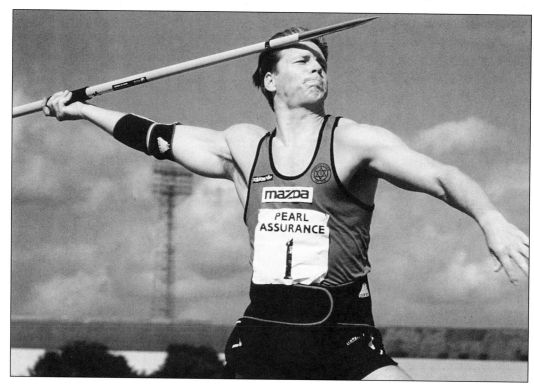

Symptoms of tenosynovitis of forearm

Symptoms of this condition include:
- Swelling and tenderness around the muscles of the forearm.
- Pain when moving the wrist and fingers.

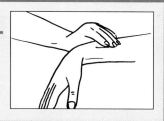

Injuries to the wrist and hand

DeQuervain's disease

Over-use of the tendons which pull the thumbs outwards produces pain and swelling over the outer side of the wrist (when the hand is facing forwards). It is commonly found in pastimes which involve rapid movements of the thumb, such as when manipulating computer games. If **RICE** fails to relieve the problem a steroid injection into the inflamed sheath of the tendon will usually effect a cure.

Fractures of the wrist

A fall onto the hand or wrist can fracture both the bones of the forearm and the small bones within the wrist. An X-ray is required to confirm the diagnosis, and they require treatment with plaster immobilization for four to six weeks.

One important small bone in the wrist is the scaphoid, which, if fractured, tends not to repair and causes chronic pain if it is not properly immobilized. For this reason persisting pain in the wrist always requires an X-ray and medical treatment.

Fractures of the hand

These are usually obvious with deformity following injury. If the injured player can be dissuaded from playing sport, treatment may simply be a case of taping two fingers together. A medical opinion should be sought at all times, however, to exclude permanent deformity.

Mallet finger

An injury to the finger tip may rupture the tendon which straightens the end of a finger

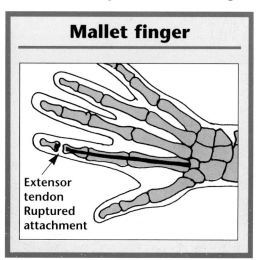

Mallet finger

Extensor
tendon
Ruptured
attachment

Upper body injuries

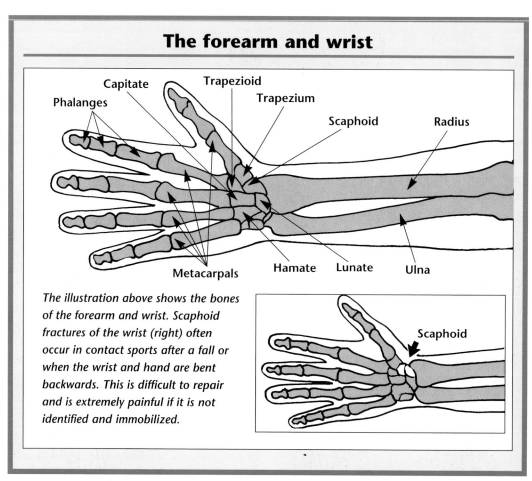

The forearm and wrist

Capitate

Phalanges

Trapezioid

Trapezium

Scaphoid

Radius

Metacarpals

Hamate

Lunate

Ulna

The illustration above shows the bones of the forearm and wrist. Scaphoid fractures of the wrist (right) often occur in contact sports after a fall or when the wrist and hand are bent backwards. This is difficult to repair and is extremely painful if it is not identified and immobilized.

Scaphoid

with the result that it cannot be fully extended. If this occurs the player must wear a splint for six weeks to enable the ruptured tendon to rejoin the bone before active mobilization is encouraged.

Sprains to digits

Where thumbs and fingers are wrenched backwards in contact sports there may be a strain of the capsule, which can be so painful as to mimic a break. Once a fracture is excluded, treatment consists of active immobilization when it is safe to do so, but strapping whenever the digit is in a situation of risk from further injury. The advice of a doctor and physiotherapist should always be sought in treatment and mobilization to prevent later handicap.

Chapter four

Backache and frontache

Backache is universal and is no more common in the sportsman than the layman, though it may be associated with many sports. Where excessive and uncontrolled twisting, lifting and contact are concerned, low back pain may be the result.

Posture

The sloucher frequently develops backache whether or not he plays sport, and any player with non-specific yet recurrent backache should seek medical and physiotherapy advice. By learning to stand and sit properly, possibly with a lumbar and thigh support,

and education in the correct and incorrect methods of lifting, backache may be alleviated if not eliminated.

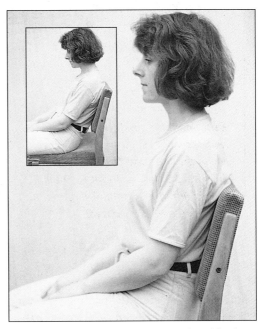

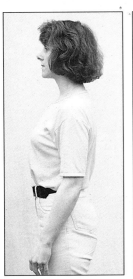
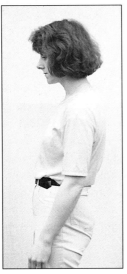

Here you can see examples of good and bad posture. Don't slump your shoulders and stick your stomach out; this puts strain on your back and may lead to backache. Instead you should stand up straight with your shoulders back and stomach pulled in. When you sit down, make sure that you sit up straight and that your back is well supported.

Backache and frontache

Slipped disc

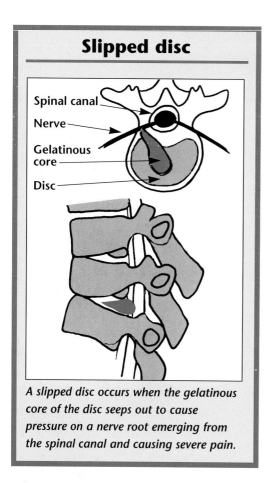

Spinal canal
Nerve
Gelatinous core
Disc

A slipped disc occurs when the gelatinous core of the disc seeps out to cause pressure on a nerve root emerging from the spinal canal and causing severe pain.

The vertebrae of the spine

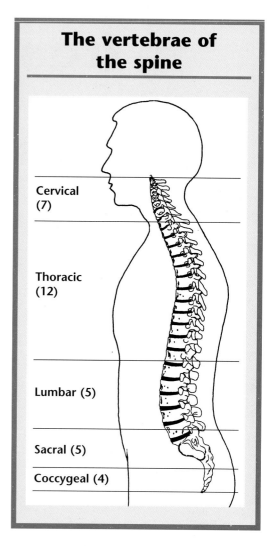

Cervical (7)

Thoracic (12)

Lumbar (5)

Sacral (5)

Coccygeal (4)

Slipped disc

Sudden backache is as likely to be due to a ligament tear or muscle spasm as to a slipped disc in which the inner gelatinous core of the flattened disc between vertebral bones seeps out to cause pressure on a nerve root emerging from the spinal canal. Sudden backache should be assumed to be from this cause until proved otherwise. The game must be stopped and the sufferer made to lie down in a comfortable position.

Sciatica

This is the pain which radiates down the leg as a result of a slipped disc and the psoas position may be found to be most comfortable. Back injuries need assessment to find a cause, though fifty per cent of back pains will get better within a week in spite of

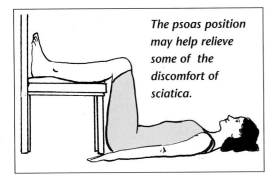

The psoas position may help relieve some of the discomfort of sciatica.

medical help with bedrest and anti-inflammatory drugs! Recurrent or continuing pains need full assessment, including X-rays and scans if appropriate, and a planned mobilization with a physiotherapist. Those that fail to resolve may need traction, manipulation or even surgery.

Sacro-iliac pain

It would seem that many sportsmen suffer pain in the joint which joins the spine to the pelvis. These sacro-iliac joints, one each side of the sacral bone, are four inches long and have a small degree of movement. It is not clear whether the pain occurs in the ligaments, which hold it together, or within the joint itself, but pain may often be felt in the buttock or the top or the back of the thigh. Where disease (ankylosing spondylitis) is not involved it is often the result of poor hip and lower back flexibility, and the pain from this area can often be eliminated if hip flexion and lumbar extension exercises are used.

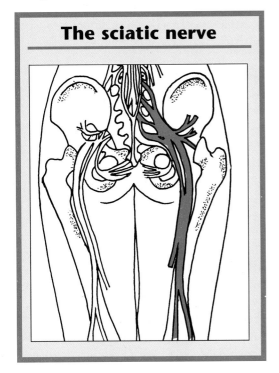

The sciatic nerve

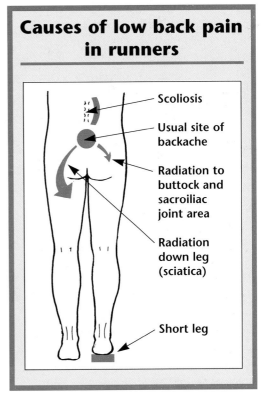

Causes of low back pain in runners

- Scoliosis
- Usual site of backache
- Radiation to buttock and sacroiliac joint area
- Radiation down leg (sciatica)
- Short leg

Backache and frontache

Groin pain

This is a common complaint of the sportsman, though the cause may not necessarily be due to sporting activity.

Swollen lymph nodes in the groin may be due to infection in the lower limb which can produce painful gland swelling either side. Naturally this needs early treatment, almost certainly with antibiotics, which are only prescribable by a doctor.

Other forms of groin pain are frequently difficult to differentiate, but the following conditions should all be considered.

Hernia

Herniae are the result of a weakness in the lower abdominal wall. In obvious cases this allows part of the abdominal organs to balloon through a narrow opening and cause groin swelling, famous for being worsened by coughing. As this can become trapped it may need urgent surgical treatment.

Sports hernia

More recently it is recognised that sportsmen suffer from a sports hernia. In this case the muscle is not so weak as to allow local ballooning, but may still require surgical repair to ease the pain.

Adductor muscle pain

The adductor muscles pull the thigh together and can be torn in sports where a sideways stretch is employed or which involve kicking a ball with the inside of the foot. Pain will be felt at the top of the groin if the sufferer attempts to hold his knees together with his legs straight whilst the examiner attempts to part them. It is usually the result of an inflexibility of the hip joint and after treatment with rest and ice, gentle stretching should be employed to ease the scarred tissue apart.

Hip disease

The older sportsman may experience pain in the groin which is in fact referred from the hip. If this appears likely the hip should be X-rayed and lack of flexibility is usually observed on examination. Physiotherapy may help mobilize this to a certain extent, but the development of severe arthritis invariably requires a hip replacement operation. After this the patient is normally advised not to pursue sports which require weight bearing and strain to be put upon the hip such as running, football or racket sports.

Osteitis pubis

A cause of severe pain in the centre of the groin is due to an instability at the meeting of the two pubic bones. This is common in footballers or where the pelvis is tilted, such as when the legs are of unequal length – a not uncommon occurrence. With prolonged rest the condition may settle, but all too frequently, even with steroid injections and physiotherapy, the player is left handicapped.

Trochanteric bursa

Pain over the outside of the hip joint may be due to an inflammation of the bursa that overlies it. Over-use or trauma will cause pain, especially if the sufferer tries to force the straightened leg outwards against resistance.

Chapter five

Leg injuries

The upper leg

There are three main groups of muscles that move the upper leg: the quadriceps at the front, the hamstrings posteriorly and the adductors on the inside of the thigh, which produce inward movement.

Quadriceps muscle tear

There is usually sudden pain which occurs when sprinting or kicking a heavy ball, and this produces local tenderness to touch. It can be tested by opposing knee straightening. The tear may be either complete when a gap can be felt between the two halves with swelling each side, in which case RICE should be used before muscle training and strengthening begins.

Where the tear is partial, again RICE should be used with physiotherapy and a steady return to training. This is likely to take two or three weeks.

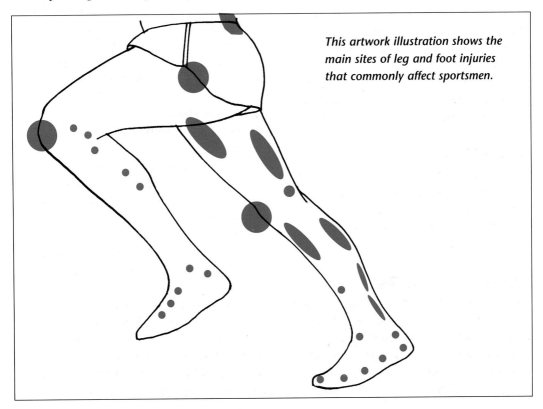

This artwork illustration shows the main sites of leg and foot injuries that commonly affect sportsmen.

Leg injuries

Hamstring tear

This usually occurs during sprinting and the sufferer has pain between the lower buttock and the knee. Stretching the muscle when bending forward with the knee straight will produce discomfort. If the tear is central there will be considerable pain but with little bruising to show for it, whereas if the tear occurs in the periphery of the muscle group, there will be visible bleeding and discolouration with much less pain. Treatment must be by RICE followed by gentle and graduated stretching. If the injury occurs at the top of the hamstring, the stretches should be performed in a different manner to that occurring in the lower half. Here the physiotherapist has to reach deep structures, which do not respond well to treatment. Hamstring tears frequently occur in conjunction with sacro-iliac discomfort and inflexibility of the lower spine so treatment must also be geared to mobilizing these structures. Many sportsmen stretch their

Hamstring strains

Hamstring strains may be caused by 'clawing' up a slope when running. Tears usually happen during sprinting and cause considerable pain.

hamstrings by toe-touching exercises. Not only does this stretch both ends of the hamstring group at once, tending to make them tear in the middle, but may also be the cause of lower back pain, and should be avoided. It is important not to treat the initial injury within a thigh muscle too ambitiously as this is frequently the site of myositis ossificans.

Hamstring exercises

These tend to be neglected in favour of quadriceps, but should be performed, and are vital if the player had an anterior cruciate injury that has not been repaired. A strong hamstring can perform the work of the anterior cruciate ligament and sometimes compensate for its absence.

Hamstring strengthening exercise

Lie face down and slowly bend your knee until the lower leg is vertical, then slowly lower to extend the leg. Repeat this slowly and frequently using a boot or small weight as the hamstrings become stronger. At home the exercise may be performed by tying the inner tube of a bicycle tyre to a solid object and looping the other end around the ankle, which gives an increasing resistance. The exercise may also be performed standing, making sure that you hold on to a solid support.

Knee injuries

In its most basic anatomy the knee is simply the junction of two sticks set one upon the other. They are held in place by collateral ligaments at the sides, which allow motion to and fro. Cruciate ligaments pass through the centre of the joint, crossing each other to prevent the lower leg bone, the tibia, moving backwards and forwards. Finally the cartilages or menisci, which are half moon-shaped pads around the sides of the joint, allow a small degree of rotation, essential if one is to turn corners! The insertions of the muscles of the upper leg surround the knee, the quadriceps being inserted into the patella or kneecap, which is simply a pulley which moves in a groove at the bottom of the upper leg bone (femur) before the patellar tendon transfers its pull to a point at the top of the tibia. The hamstring group split above and behind the knee to be inserted into areas each side of the knee, and it is the triple pull exerted by these groups of muscles that provides the stability that the knee requires to prevent collapse. If one of the muscle groups is weak, instability is more likely with resultant injury to the knee. By following this elementary anatomy it should be easier to understand the injuries that occur.

Effusion

A knee swollen by blood or clear serous fluid is said to contain an effusion and will be painful to move outside a narrow range. A rapid effusion of the knee, especially following trauma or twisting, has a seventy per cent

likelihood of being caused by a ruptured cruciate ligament, usually the anterior one. Whilst this should be treated with first aid by **RICE**, urgent medical assessment is required to drain off the fluid and, if necessary, arthroscope or perform surgery to repair the ligament. Full flexibility of the joint will need to be obtained before strength training begins.

Pre-patellar bursa (housemaid's knee)

This superficial swelling over the front of the kneecap usually occurs as the result of direct trauma or kneeling for too long. If ice and anti-inflammatory drugs do not settle the condition, it may prove necessary to drain the fluid and inject with cortisone to avoid surgery.

Arthritis

Older players with wear and tear in this joint may attempt to play sport, and swelling and pain within the knee joint may be the result. Rest, warmth, anti-inflammatory drugs, physiotherapy and cortisone injections may all slow the wear and tear process for some time, but invariably the player either has to desist from most active sport or risk the need for a knee replacement. Exercise which avoids weight bearing, such as cycling or swimming, can be sustained for much longer than those that involve impact with a hard surface.

Meniscus tear

Any of the cartilages may be torn in various ways if sudden twisting movements are

Leg injuries

performed, though the medial ones are most commonly affected. This may result in locking of the knee or increasing pain as the knee is slowly fully extended. Cartilage only has a small ability to heal itself so to prevent the loose flap causing further damage to cartilage attached to the bone within the joint, it is now customary to remove the damaged areas at arthroscopy. This operation involves a small cut in the skin to the side of the knee through which a fibre-optic scope is passed enabling the surgeon to visualize the interior of this or any other joint. By further insertion of small instruments, dead or damaged tissue may be removed. Following this the knee must be fully mobilized before sport is attempted.

Hoffar's syndrome

Many sportsmen, particularly runners, are concerned by pain and swelling which can occur below each side of the kneecap. This is fat rather than fluid and occurs following over-use. It is one of the causes of anterior knee pain and is normally settled using RICE, anti-inflammatories, physiotherapy and occasionally a cortisone injection. The player should reduce his training to the amount that was comfortable before the condition occurred.

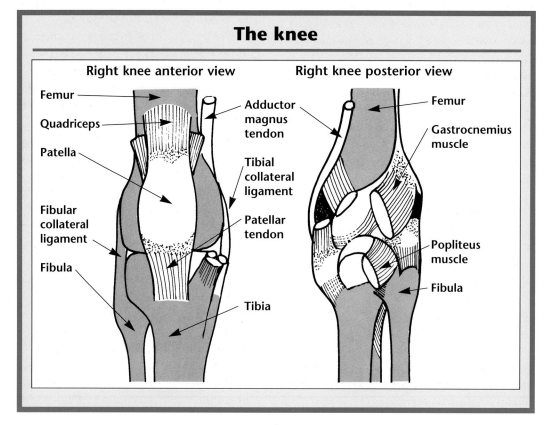

The knee

Right knee anterior view

Femur
Quadriceps
Patella
Fibular collateral ligament
Fibula

Adductor magnus tendon
Tibial collateral ligament
Patellar tendon
Tibia

Right knee posterior view

Femur
Gastrocnemius muscle
Popliteus muscle
Fibula

Baker's cyst

A weakness of the capsule or lining of the knee joint may allow a herniation to produce a fluid swelling behind the knee known as a Baker's cyst. Most concern about this condition is due to its appearance, but if it enlarges or becomes tender it may require surgical removal.

Locking knees

Although a torn cartilage may cause locking of knees, they also become solidly locked if a piece of loose bone or cartilage prevents normal flexion or extension of the knee. Osteochondritis dissecans is a condition which can particularly affect young footballers where trauma causes fragments to break off from the articular surface of the bones to float about within the joint causing pain and disability. The diagnosis can be confirmed by X-ray. It is sometimes possible to surgically re-attach the loose body, but as osteoarthritis is more prevalent in sportsmen who have suffered from osteochondritis dissecans they are advised to reduce their sporting activity.

Anterior knee pain

A large number of sports players complain of aching and pain at front of the knee. Not all of this is necessarily due to serious injury, but may be the result of a combination of minor wear to the posterior surface of the patella and to imbalances in the strength of the muscles that control it. The pain which is so common, and can be severe enough to prevent the player from running or participating in sport, may well be due to some obvious injury, but all too often no trauma has occurred and with an absence of swelling or deformity there may be little evidence that the knee is at all different to the other. However, subtle variations can be established which make the difference between discomfort and pleasure from sport.

Chondromalacia patellae

This name is sometimes used to describe the condition where the kneecap fails to move smoothly in the groove at the bottom of the upper leg bone where it acts as a pulley allowing the knee to be straightened. It is important to remember that when we stand still with our heels together the knees are also close to each other while the hips are separated by upward of one foot. This means that the further above the knee one is, the further the thighs and thigh muscles are separated, and therefore pull at a slight angle upon their insertions around the knee, which can have painful consequences. The quadriceps muscles are inserted into the top of the patella and have a wide spread over the front of the thigh. Should the pull through these groups be unequal, the patella will tend to be deviated towards one side, usually the outer, with the result that it rubs painfully in the patellar groove causing in some cases a persistent aching and in others such an acute pain that the sportsman is forced to stop sport immediately. It may exist as a primary condition or as the secondary effect of a previous injury to the knee or quadriceps which disturbs the pull of this muscle group.

One part of the quadriceps mechanism is the muscle on the inside of the thigh which only contracts fully when the knee is

Leg injuries

straightened and locked in full extension. If this muscle is not used or is over-powered by sportsmen developing the outer quadriceps to its detriment, the sheer tone and power of the outer muscles may induce the condition. Thus bent knee exercise, such as performing squats or lifting heavy weights, may cause a relative weakness of the inner muscles and be sufficient to make the condition occur. Similarly running hard downhill, which is controlled by sudden quadriceps contraction, can cause the posterior surface of the patella to be bruised against the femoral groove and produce a similar pain. The imbalance must be reduced by performing straight leg quadriceps exercises (below).

Physiotherapy may also help, but as the condition often affects young gymnasts, teenage girls and young women, if they suffer from this condition they may have to alter the way they sit on the ground on their haunches with their knees tightly flexed underneath. Similarly anyone suffering from anterior knee pain would do well to try to learn to stand with their knees braced, working the inner quadriceps muscles rather than slouching with knees bent. Some players with chondromalacia patellae find the condition so painful that they subject themselves to surgery, but the results of this are not particularly encouraging and concentration on straight knee exercises will usually cure the problem if they are persevered with.

Straight leg quadriceps exercises

Lying down on your back with your legs straight and toes flexed, bend the foot of the injured leg upwards. Lift the leg off the floor, keeping the knee straight. Hold for a count of 10, then lower the leg to the floor and rest it for 10 seconds. Do 10 repetitions.

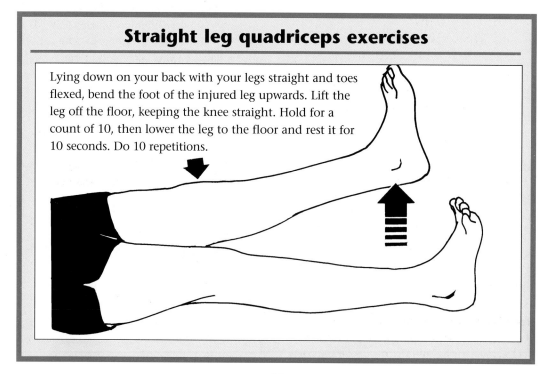

Jumper's knee

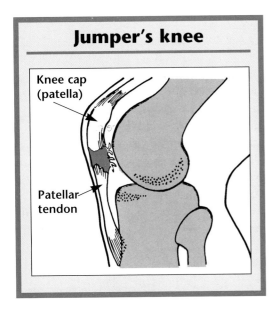

Knee cap (patella)

Patellar tendon

Patellar tendinitis

The small tendon between patella and the top of the lower leg bone (the tibia) has all the forces of the quadriceps muscles pulling through it. As such it is prone to tendinitis or partial tears, which occur particularly at the back of the tendon just where it leaves the patella. This is often known as 'jumper's knee'. It is frequently caused by overloading when jumping or when taking off on one leg. Whilst rest, ice and physiotherapy may help, the injured player will almost certainly have to reduce the amount of exercise he performs. It can be resistant to treatment and on occasion cortisone injections or even surgery may be required.

Osgood Schlatter's disease

Many teenage boys complain of pain below the knee with a swelling at the upper end of the tibia into which the patellar tendon is inserted. This form of disease is known as osteochondritis and is named after Drs. Osgood and Schlatter. It is an over-use injury of the growing point in which pain and inflammation occur. It was always customary to ban boys with this condition from sport, but it is now considered more relevant to allow them to play some games within the limit of their pain. If there is any doubt about the diagnosis the knee should be X-rayed and then the player encouraged to treat it whenever sore with ice packs and mild anti-inflammatory drugs until it has recovered enough to allow play. As a word of warning, no child should be allowed to play whilst the medicine is in their system in case it masks further injury. The condition almost invariably cures itself with time and very few children find a lengthy restriction from exercise to be needed, although in the unlucky ones it may linger through their teenage years.

Osgood Schlatter's knee

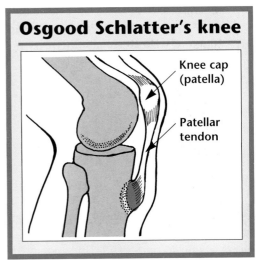

Knee cap (patella)

Patellar tendon

Leg injuries

Other knee conditions

Ligament strains

By accident or design in some sports pressure may be exerted on the outside or the inside of the knee attempting to force it laterally. This stresses either the medial or lateral collateral ligaments, which allow the hinge movement forwards and backwards through which the knee moves. This type of injury may cause swelling and there will certainly be pain, usually enough to make the sufferer limp. As these ligaments are vital for knee stability, it is important they are allowed to heal properly once diagnosis has been made by a doctor. RICE is highly important and whilst healing of the ligament occurs the muscles which stabilise the knee must be trained to prevent the knee being accidentally moved sideways and the ligament retorn.

The exercises needed are the same straight leg exercises as were used for rehabilitating after chondromalacia patellae (see page 64) and further emphasises the need for strong thigh muscles to stabilize the knee. Once the training exercises are started the strength of the knee should be regularly tested by a doctor or physiotherapist, and full rehabilitation must have taken place before any competition whatsoever is allowed.

Ilio-tibial friction band syndrome

As well as the muscles which stabilise the knee there is a sheet of rough muscular tissue running down the outside of the leg known as the ilio-tibial band. This normally rides without friction over the outer side of the lower end of the femur, but if sportsmen are at all bow-legged this band may rub against the bony prominence causing a clicking discomfort when the knee is slightly bent, though it does not occur when the knee is fully straightened. It may be possible to correct the gait with shoe build-ups to prevent the exaggerated bow-leggedness, but some sportsmen require steroid injections between bone and ilio-tibial tract if ice and physiotherapy fail to settle the condition.

Exercise used in the treatment of knee injuries

Before exercises to build up the power of the thigh muscles are used the sportsman should firstly endeavour to ensure that it bends and extends to the same degree as easily as the other knee. The exercises may then be commenced, attempting to maintain a balance of power between the muscle groups. The inner quadriceps muscles only tighten firmly when the knee is locked straight. You can test this yourself. As a result certain exercises to build up the quadriceps, such as leg extension machines, may build up the outer quadriceps muscles to the detriment of the inner ones, especially if the knee is not fully extended.

Lower leg injuries

Stress fractures

The most common sites of stress fractures are one third of the way from knee to ankle in both the tibia and fibula. It is usually caused by sudden changes in training patterns, but will require six weeks or so of rest from pain provoking activity to fully recover. A small proportion fail to heal and may require surgical treatment. Stress fractures may be tested by a competent physiotherapist using an ultrasound test. This sets up an unpleasant discomfort in the cracked ends and is often of value in persuading the dubious sportsman of the need to rest!

Shin splints

This is an imprecise term referring to pain within the tibia. However, as well as stress fractures there are two other major causes that need to be differentiated.

Anterior compartment syndrome

The muscles of the lower leg are enclosed within tight inelastic sheaths in three major groups. That at the front outer side is known as the anterior compartment. An increase in training or change of playing surface may cause the muscles to overwork, swell and become more tightly enclosed within this compartment. It can usually be treated with RICE and anti-inflammatory drugs and physiotherapy. Orthotics may also help, but the player must be advised to alter his training more gradually. The lateral and posterior compartments may also be affected in a similar way, though usually less severely as their sheaths bind the muscles less tightly.

Tibial periostitis

Many sportsmen, particularly those who run, complain of pain on the inner side of the lower tibia, worsened by exercise. If compartment syndromes and stress fracture have been eliminated as a diagnosis, it may well be due to the muscle originating from the bone being pulled away to cause a painful periosteal inflammation. It is particularly common in those who pronate (see page 72) or who suffer from a dropped longitudinal foot arch. If RICE and stretching fail to resolve the pain quite dramatic recoveries can be obtained by raising the arch with an orthotic device to alter the stance and gait of the player.

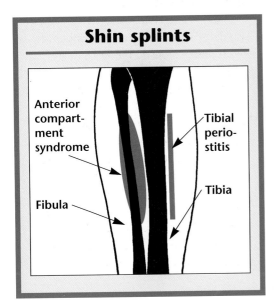

Shin splints

Anterior compart-ment syndrome

Fibula

Tibial perio-stitis

Tibia

Leg injuries

Calf strains

The two major calf muscles may frequently be torn, especially if there is sudden awkward uncontrolled movement of the ankle causing the heel to drop. The player will complain of sudden pain, especially noticeable when attempting to stand on his toes or to stretch forward with heels to the ground. Treatment should be with RICE for 48 hours before gentle stretching is commenced. Over the course of three or four weeks this must be increased until calf movements are painless and as full as in the other ankle, before strengthening is commenced. To achieve this the player should stand with the ball of his foot on a stair and as slowly as possible raise and lower the heel. When the power in the

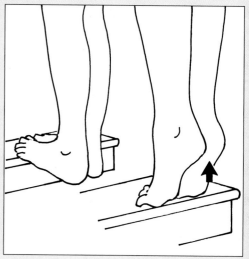

injured calf is equal to that of the other leg, training and competition may commenced.

Achilles tendon

The achilles tendon joins the calf muscle to the heel bone (calcaneum) but it has a very poor blood supply and so it may be injured in various ways.

Ruptured achilles tendon

This can break with an audible snap. The player is unable to stand on tiptoe and there is swelling, discomfort and a palpable gap between the split ends of the tendon. Treatment is required if the player is to walk let alone compete again and surgery is

usually the favoured method, though some surgeons prefer to put the ankle in plaster and allow it to heal whilst immobile. Full achilles mobilization must be completed before any competition is contemplated.

Achilles tendinitis

There is often pain following exercise. The tendon does not swell, but can be painful to touch. Rest and ice will ease the condition, because if it is neglected it invariably becomes chronic.

Achilles peritendinitis

This particular tendon has a surrounding paratenon, which may itself become inflamed, sometimes following untreated tendinitis as described above. There is visible swelling and movement of the tendon as the ankle is gently flexed and extended may produce a sensation known as crepitus, a sort of crackling under the fingers examining the tendon. The condition may be caused by unsuitable shoes (see opposite) and this may be one of the few instances when a steroid injection is of value around the achilles.

Partial rupture of achilles tendon

Frequently the only findings with achilles pain are one or more little tender nicks on the outer or inner side of the tendon. These represent a small partial rupture which not only heals badly owing to the poor blood supply but also heals 'short' as most humans tend to sleep with their toes pointed and with the injured area unstretched through the night. When the patient first gets out of bed to walk in the morning the tendon is immediately stretched as the heel hits the ground and causes the patient considerable discomfort for the first ten minutes or so as the injured area is re-stretched and frequently re-torn.

Other causes of heel pain

Calcaneal bursa Between the achilles and the heel bone into which the tendon is inserted (the calcaneus) lies a bursa. This can be inflamed by uncomfortable shoes which rub against the heel to produce a form of deep blistering. As a result there is redness, heat

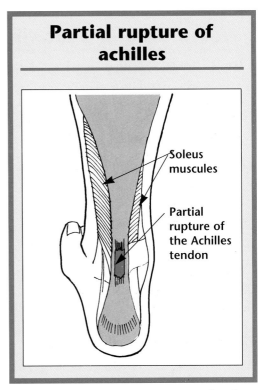

Partial rupture of achilles

Soleus muscules

Partial rupture of the Achilles tendon

and swelling. The bursa can be treated with RICE, anti-inflammatory tablets and physiotherapy, but if ignored or neglected may result in the player requiring a cortisone injection or even surgery.

In many cases it may be possible to prevent calcaneal bursitis occurring by ensuring that new shoes are properly and slowly worn in or by stretching the heel of a shoe which has previously initiated the pain. The rubbing may be prevented if vertical strips of orthopaedic felt or foam are placed inside the shoe at points that will not impinge upon the bursa. The condition occurs as a result of friction, so this should be avoided within the heel area of the shoe.

Leg injuries

Prevention and treatment of achilles tendon injuries

Shoes Many shoes possess a high heel tab which digs into the achilles tendon at the site of injury. This may bruise it more than one thousand times per mile run. All of this heel tab should be excised horizontally apart from the inner layer, which is usually made of a thin artificial material, which can be turned over the back of the shoes and stuck down with some form of superglue. Despite fears to the contrary, shoes treated like this fall off no more easily than untreated footwear!

Heel raises If the heels are slightly raised within the shoe the achilles tendon is similarly shortened and less prone to injury from sudden lengthening. The raise may be achieved either by persuading a cobbler to insert a wedge of rubbery material between the base of the shoe and the mid-sole, or by placing one of the formed rubber wedges which are available from drugstores under the heel. Both achieve the same aim.

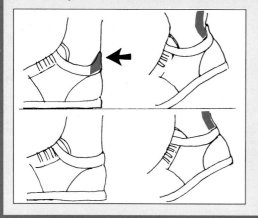

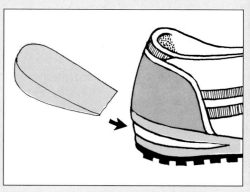

The ankle

Although the ankle may appear to be a simple mortice joint which permits movement forwards and backwards, there is also a lower joint which permits rotational movement of the foot from side to side. By using the small muscles of the foot with those that strap the ankle we are able to balance when standing still. The initial movement allows plantar flexion (downward) and dorsi flexion (upward) movement, and the lower joint permits inversion (inward) and eversion (outward) movement.

Ankle sprain

This common injury can occur throughout life but is more common in sportsmen who slip or play on an uneven surface. The majority of injuries involve inversion so that the three ligaments that join the fibula to the talus, the bone enclosed by the mortice, become wrenched and one or more may totally or partially rupture. It causes considerable pain, worsened when the foot is moved inwards, and there may be visible bruising to the outside of the foot. It may be impossible to differentiate this injury from a fracture unless an X-ray is performed.

At first treatment must be by RICE, avoidance of weight bearing in the severe cases and use of crutches before gentle mobilization is attempted after 48 hours. Severe cases require strapping, but the benefits of this must be weighed against the consequent disuse of the ankle strap muscles, which are required to provide stability and strength during recovery. Initially the player should aim to increase the range of movement, always comparing the injured ankle with the uninjured. Once mobility has been obtained the injured player should walk about in bare feet alternately on heels and toes, then the insides and outsides of the feet. Strength can be obtained by standing on a lower stair and performing calf strengthening exercises and also by performing step exercises.

One vital loss with an inversion sprain is proprioception – the ability to know where you are in space. To recover this attempt to stand with eyes closed on the injured leg alone. If you think you are good, compare the time that you can manage on that leg with the uninjured one. One excellent method of recovery from all lower limb injuries is by the use of a wobble board

The usual ankle strain involves damage to the ligaments on the outside of the joint. Occasionally those within the joint may be affected and bleeding takes place into the ankle joint itself – a haemarthrosis. It is possible to differentiate between the two types of sprain by observing the ankle from behind and looking to see whether one or both hollows to the side of the achilles tendon are filled out. One suggests an external sprain, both a haemarthrosis. The haemarthrosis caused by an internal sprain will require more physiotherapy and time before healing is complete.

If the lateral ankle ligaments are completely ruptured rather than simply torn there is a risk of a permanently unstable ankle. Careful physiotherapy and mobilization may heal it satisfactorily, but occasionally surgery is required to effect a cure for this injury.

A sprained ankle is probably the most poorly treated sports injury generally.

Footballer's ankle

Multiple trauma and kicking impacts at the front of the ankle may cause repeated strain and inflammation. As a result little bony osteophytes may develop within the ankle joint and limit its range of movement with increased pain. The footballer will need to cease play and possibly subject himself to surgery to prevent chronic pain from a young age.

Chapter six

Foot injuries

Common injuries to the back of the heel have been dealt with in the achilles tendon section, but the rim and underneath of the heel, as well as the bony and muscular structures of the foot, are particularly prone to sporting injury.

Heel angle pain

Sporting youngsters may suffer from an osteochondritis (like Osgood Schlatter's disease) of the heel, known as Sever's disease. The pulling tendon is usually too painful to permit running or jumping though with RICE and heel padding some activity may be possible. This area may also be affected in the older runner due to some traction by the achilles insertion, but this can also be confused with bruising of the heel caused by frequent impact. The bruising may be helped by fitting a heel cup, which condenses the fat pad under the heel, the increased thickness making it more able to absorb trauma. Performance of gentle Achilles tendon stretches regularly will also help to prevent and eliminate the problem.

Foot structure

Each step we take involves a complex series of movements within the foot from heel strike to take-off. On landing the foot is turned slightly in so the outer border receives the impact, only to rotate outwardly to allow the flat of the foot and maximum surface area to be in contact with the ground in mid-stance. As take-off occurs the foot again rotates slightly inwards until it regains its original position. The word supination describes the position where the underside of the foot is turned in and pronation describes the movement outwards. The average person has a mildly supinated foot with a longitudinal arch present between the ball of the foot and the heel. This is exaggerated in pes cavus (high arch). With flat feet (pes planus) the foot is more pronated.

Pronation is the more common of the two and its presence may lead to a predisposition towards many of the conditions already discussed. Amongst these are low back and hip pain, anterior knee pain, compartment syndromes and tibial periostitis,

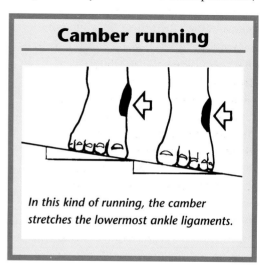

Camber running

In this kind of running, the camber stretches the lowermost ankle ligaments.

Pronation

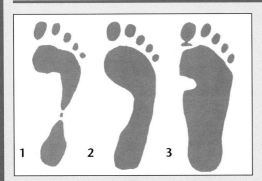

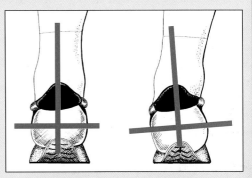

Above: These three illustrations show: 1 The footprint of a runner with a high instep (pes cavus); 2 The footprint of a normal foot; and 3 The footprint of a flat-footed runner with increased pronation.

Above: When a runner pronates(right), the foot and shoe tilt inwards which may lead to injury, especially in the shins and knees. Good shoes, special inserts and orthotics can help prevent and alleviate the problem.

Achilles tendon problems due to the shearing stresses involved within the tendon itself, and some foot problems to be discussed in this chapter. Pronation may also be exaggerated if a sportsman possesses the not uncommon problem that legs are of different lengths, or are made artificially so by running persistently on uneven camber. It may be possible to treat pronation induced injury by the use of suitable orthotics or orthoses. These are shoe inserts that can be precisely or approximately made to the contour of the underside of the athletes foot, the cheapest and least reliable being made from home-made foam rubber cut-outs, the most precise and most expensive, those that are made from a plaster of Paris negative impression of the sportsman's foot. Rigid orthoses are sometimes supplied, which appear adequate for the non-

sportsman, but which many players find uncomfortable. The orthotic should, therefore, have some flexibility and be able to fit in the sportsman's shoe without causing tightness or discomfort. Sometimes the effect of an orthotic is little short of miraculous: for other players they may take longer to wear in.

Plantar fasciitis

As in the palm of the hand, the foot also has a fascia which bowstrings between the front of the heel bone (calcaneus) and the front of the long foot bones (metatarsals). If this is over-stretched as a result of competing on hard surfaces or in stiff footwear or even in the non-sportsman with flat-feet, acute pain and irritation occurs at its origin. Diagnosis should be simple. There is acute pain on pressing at the front of the calcaneus and the

Foot injuries

sportsman will find that he cannot play through it. Conservative treatment should be with physiotherapy and an orthotic arch support, and the use of anti-inflammatory tablets. Doctors are inclined to treat this with a cortisone injection, but are not invariably successful, hence the need for other treatments.

Metatarsalgia

Many sportsmen develop pain at the toe end of their metatarsal bones where the ligaments become strained. Just as the foot has a longitudinal arch, so it also has a transverse raised arch at this level, and patients with metatarsalgia may well develop callouses underneath as a result of a dropped arch. The arch may be reformed to a certain extent by exercises for the small muscles of the feet or by physiotherapy with faradic currents to stimulate the muscles into action. However, most players require a metatarsal arch support placed centrally just behind the heads of the metatarsal, which alter the pressure points and fulcrum for take-off.

Morton's neuroma

This term is used to describe the swelling of a nerve between the third and fourth metatarsal heads in a dropped anterior arch, which causes acute pain at the site, but often with an associated numbness of the adjacent sides of the appropriate toes. Relief from tight shoes may ease the problem as may a metatarsal arch support, which lifts and separates metatarsal heads. However, failing this, cortisone injections and surgery may well be required.

Hallux rigidus

Pain at the junction between the first metatarsal and the big toe may well be due to immobility as the result of premature arthritis. Any attempt on examination to stretch the toe through its full range induces sharp pains. It may be associated with plantar fasciitis. Initially the condition can be relieved with the use of anti-inflammatory drugs and self-help physiotherapy to enlarge the range of movement. Padding in the shoe or a softer landing surface may help, but altering the fulcrum by means of a metatarsal bar behind the heads of the bones may again relieve the condition, provided the sportsman's shoe is not too overcrowded! Resistant cases may eventually require surgery, though the loss of leverage may severely handicap the competitive player.

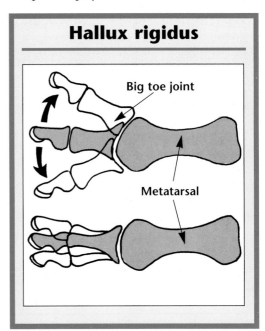

Hallux rigidus

Big toe joint

Metatarsal

Other medical problems

Cramp

Cramp is characterized by a localized muscle spasm during or after exercise. It is usually related to tiredness and water or electrolyte depletion or imbalance. It is less common in the well trained, but if it persists further medical investigations should be carried out. It is usually possible to treat the acute attack by a passive stretch of the affected muscle and release of any tight clothing such as socks or belts. The onset may be delayed if sufficient fluid is drunk during competition.

Athlete's foot

This fungal skin infection tends to commence with irritation between the fourth and fifth toes which spread to the underside and other sweaty areas of the feet. It is more common if the player sweats heavily as will occur with unwashed socks or shoes with an upper surface that cannot breathe. If it fails to clear with foot and clothing hygiene, anti-fungal creams and powders will usually resolve the infection.

Stitch

The pain felt with stitch is usually a spasm of the dome-like diaphragm, the muscle which divides chest from abdomen. There is no one cause, but may well follow or occur during unaccustomed eating or exercise. It is less common in the well trained sportsman and is provoked by eating or drinking too close to competition. Ideally there should be a three-hour gap between eating with the sportsman drinking small quantities of water in the interval period prior to starting exercise.

The spasm can sometimes be abolished if the player takes in a deep breath and holds it for as long as is comfortable or practises a few trunk flexions whilst on the move. If its frequency increases a full medical examination should be instigated.

Blisters

No player is immune from blisters at all times, usually affecting either feet or hands. They are more common in hot or humid conditions and when using new equipment, clothing or footwear. Fluid builds up between two layers of skin as a result of friction and although medical opinion is divided, they seem to heal quicker if burst with a sterile needle and the overlying areas of dead skin are allowed to harden and protect the underlying structures.

Many sportsmen like to prevent rubbing by using petroleum jelly or talc, or to harden the skin by rubbing it with surgical spirit regularly. Where an acute blister occurs in competition, a second skin material may prevent it worsening.

Chapter seven

Injuries by sport

Running

This is the most basic of sports involving the lower limbs and tends to involve movement in a reasonably straight line. Because of the high knee lift in sprinting, the injury patterns are different to those found in long distance running.

Distance running injuries

Owing to stiff upright styles many distance runners complain of low back pain. This can be eased with lumbar extension exercises and hip flexion. Runner's knee is particularly common in the slower distance runner who may benefit from increasing his speed and exercising his inner quadriceps muscles better. Shin-splints and lower limb stress fractures may be associated with poor foot biomechanics and can often be corrected by a change in shoes or the insertion of orthotics. Variations on these may help ease many of the causes of foot pain that is found in distance runners. If achilles tendon injuries are not the result of improper shoes they need delicate treatment and rehabilitation to prevent chronic injuries occurring.

Sprinting

Coming out of the blocks or start is aided by externally rotating the legs and using adductor strength to start off. This frequently leads to adductor pulls though it is in full flight that hamstring and quadriceps tears usually occur, especially if there is a tight bend. A flexibility routine built into a training schedule may help prevent many of these injuries and competition should not be allowed until the sprinter is fluent in his stride and pain-free.

Football

The modern tendency to kick the ball with the instep rather than the toecap causes adductor strains and osteitis pubis in even well prepared footballers. The most commonly injured group of muscles is the quadriceps group, especially if a tackle is made blocking the leg extension. The twisting involved in football frequently results in a torn mensicus and ligament strains, which must be fully rehabilitated to prevent wasting of thigh muscles and ensuing instability. Osgood Schlatter's Disease is invariably found in teenage footballers who tend to develop a footballer's ankle as their skills increase and the tackling becomes heavier.

Racket sports

Light rackets (badminton, squash etc.)
Shoulder injuries are frequently found on the playing arm and over-reaching is liable to cause rotator cuff strains and a sub-acromial bursitis. Faulty grips and technique may be the cause of tenosynovitis of the forearm and tennis elbow, which can be corrected by a

good coach. The twisting involved may produce anterior cruciate and meniscal injury, while the unprepared player will always get blisters at various pressure points.

Heavy racket (tennis) The arm is held much more stiffly to control the heavier racket, which can cause painful strains of the more tautly held muscles and the fore and upper arm. The inexpert player is advised to have a light head to the racket and slightly looser stringing to cause less shock. Naturally shoulder injuries are common, as are those related to running and twisting.

Skiing

Despite the amount of protective clothing, skiing injuries are far too common. Modern bindings help to limit ankle injuries, but many serious knee problems occur, particularly affecting the ligaments and menisci. Thumbs may become particularly sore as the ligaments are stretched after prolonged use of sticks.

Hockey

Many hockey injuries are similar to those sustained in soccer as a result of the running and twisting action. However, the forward lean needed to control the stick may cause low back pain and this may also increase the number of hamstring injuries. The use of artificial turf leads to nasty burns in a fall which require first aid and cleaning.

Golf

This sport is used as exercise by many older people, but they may suffer through lack of mobility. Low back and shoulder pain will result from inflexibility, which needs to be corrected before a club is picked up. Golfer's elbow is usually due to poor technique, which should be corrected earlier in the golfer's career rather than when bad habits are established.

Cycling

Although cycling is good cardio-vascular exercise and produces none of the problems in the lower limbs related to hitting hard ground, it may well be a source of back pain, especially if the saddle is not at the correct height. An uncomfortable saddle will also produce groin pain and saddle soreness, and should be adjusted. The position of the hands on handlebars may produce carpal tunnel syndrome and ulnar nerve discomfort. Knee pain is not as common as might be expected in a sport in which the knees are not fully extended, but if present may require a change of saddle height. Falls onto hard tarmac may produce severe grazing which requires cleaning and first aid.

Rugby Union & League

These contact sports may produce a number of severe injuries. Concussion is not uncommon, especially after scrums and mauls, and there is great danger to the back and neck if a scrum collapses. Shoulder dislocations are common on hard ground and the lower limb may suffer all the injuries associated with running and twisting. Anterior cruciate ligament ruptures are particularly common amongst top class players.

Injuries by sport

Methods of treatment

Physiotherapy in its many forms is an important treatment for the injured sportsman. However, many sports players imagine it to be no more than a pleasant half hour under a heat lamp. The skilled chartered sports physiotherapist will use many different types of treatment depending on the type, age and depth of injury.

Massage This is the oldest form of physiotherapy but still has a very large part to play in treatment. It is of particular value in freeing scarred tissue, though if used over-enthusiastically can cause more damage and worsen injuries if friction is over-enthusiastically performed.

Ultrasound An ultrasound machine emits waves too high to be audible to the human ear. However, it can promote healing by stimulating local blood flow and reducing the inflammatory process.

Interferential Electrical currents are passed through the damaged area from dampened pads that are placed around the injury. The crossing of these waves stimulates and heats the area as well as providing a numbing effect.

Short wave This machine uses a high frequency current to create magnetic fields which reduce inflammation, swelling and pain by heating up the tissues.

Manipulation This is used by many medical practitioners as a method of mobilising stiffened and locked joints which do not respond to other methods. They help with joint mobility but must be used with great caution and never by an inexperienced practitioner.

Lasers The energy produced by lasers assists healing by various biochemical pathways, the local energy produced seeming to speed up the rate of healing and return to normal.

Taping Taping a limb helps to prevent abnormal movement into a position that has produced previous or unhealed injury. Taping by an expert will provide a full and painless range of movement, though its use is not to be encouraged on a regular basis owing to the weakening of muscles that results.

Anti-inflammatory drugs

There are many drugs related to aspirin which can be used as an aid to treatment. When used correctly they decrease the production of prostaglandins, chemicals which are formed after injury and produce swelling and pain. Whilst a short course may be reasonable, it is important that sportsmen should not compete or train heavily whilst taking them, for they may mask further or worsening injury.

In some people they can also have multiple side-effects and may initiate ulcers or asthma in predisposed individuals. Although some are available over the counter, they should not be taken for more than a short course without medical guidance.

Useful information

**National Sports Medicine
Institute**
St Bartholomew's Medical
College
Charterhouse Square
London EC1M 6BQ
Tel: 0171 251 0583

**British Association Sport
and Medicine**
BASM Education Officer
C/O N.S.M.I.
St Bartholomew's Medical
College
Charterhouse Square
London EC1M 6BQ
Tel: 0171 253 3244

British Olympic Association
1 Wandsworth Plain
London SW18 1EH
Tel: 0181 871 2677

Sports Council
16 Upper Woburn Place
London WC1H 0QP
Tel: 0171 388 1277

**National Coaching
Foundation**
114 Cardigan Road
Headingly
Leeds
LS6 3BJ
Tel: 0113 274 4802

British Athletics Federation
225A Bristol Road
Edgbaston
Birmingham B5 7UB
Tel: 0121 440 5000

**North Cheshire Sports
Injuries Clinic**
85 High Street
Runcorn
Cheshire WA7 1JF
Tel: 01928 561358

Overseas Organisations

Australia
Athletics Australia
PO Box 1400
North Melbourne
3051 Victoria

Canada
Athletics Canada
1600 James Naismith Drive
Gloucester
Ontario K1B SN4

New Zealand
Athletics New Zealand
PO Box 741
Wellington

South Africa
Athletics SA
PO Box 1261
Pretoria 0001

United States
**The American College of
Sports Medicine**
PO Box 1440
401 West Michigan Street
Indianapolis
Indiana 46202-3233
Tel: 317 637 9200

**The Athletics Congress of
the USA**
PO Box 120
Indianapolis
Indiana 46206-0120

Index